Keep Your Voice Healthy

Advisory Editor
William H. Perkins, Ph.D.
Professor of Communication Arts and Sciences,
Otolaryngology, and Speech Science
University of Southern California
Los Angeles, California

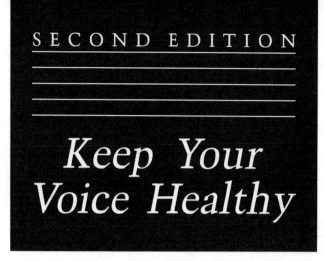

SECOND EDITION

Keep Your Voice Healthy

A Guide to the Intelligent Use and Care of the Speaking and Singing Voice

By Friedrich S. Brodnitz, M.D.

Associate Attending Otolaryngologist
Mount Sinai Medical Center
New York City
Consultant Otolaryngologist
Lenox Hill Hospital
New York City

With a Foreword by Leontyne Price

A College-Hill Publication
Little, Brown and Company
Boston/Toronto

College-Hill Press
A Division of Little, Brown and Company (Inc.)
34 Beacon Street
Boston, Massachusetts 02108

© **1988 by Little, Brown and Company (Inc.)**
First Edition published by Harper & Row in 1953; a reprint edition was published by Charles C. Thomas in 1973.

Second Printing

Library of Congress Cataloging in Publication Data

Brodnitz, Friedrich S., 1899–
   Keep your voice healthy: a guide to the intelligent use and care of the speaking and singing voice/by Friedrich S. Brodnitz; introduction by Leontyne Price. — 2nd ed.
   160 p.
   "A College-Hill publication."
   Includes index.
   ISBN 0-316-10902-9
   1. Voice — Care and hygiene.   2. Speech.   I. Title.
RF465.B75 1987
617'.533 — dc19   87-23751
                                                                    CIP
                                                                    MN

ISBN 0-316-109029

Printed in the United States of America

CONTENTS

To the memory of
Manuel Garcia *(1805–1906)*
Singer, teacher, scientist

who gave to medicine the laryngeal mirror
and opened a new era
in the study of the human voice

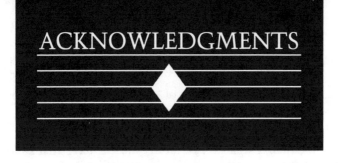

ACKNOWLEDGMENTS

To write a popular book on a medical subject is impossible without the help of a great many people.

First of all, science is, by its very nature, a cooperative undertaking. The doctor who writes for his colleagues in medical journals or books quotes his sources in numerous footnotes. In popular writing this technique would be confusing to the reader. But I want to say that all of the workers who, by their original thoughts and research, developed the science of the human voice and speech are, in a deeper sense, the co-authors of this book.

Thanks are due to my patients and to the students of my lectures and courses on voice problems who, through their questions, helped to test and clarify the terms, definitions, and explanations I had to give on many occasions. Their willingness to listen and to partake in discussions of a sometimes rather involved subject has encouraged me to write this book in nontechnical language but without the oversimplification that is the danger of popular medical literature.

A number of friends, colleagues, and scientists have helped me immensely by their generous and selfless assistance in putting this book together:

- Helmuth Nathan, M.D., of New York City, contributed drawings.
- Gordon E. Peterson, Ph.D., of Murray Hill, New Jersey, and R. R. Garcia, of New York City, both of the Bell Telephone Laboratories, supplied photographs of the vocal folds.
- Joel J. Pressman, M.D., of Beverly Hills, California (and the American Medical Association as publishers) permitted the use of illustrations from his paper on the vocal folds in the *Archives of Otolaryngology*, 1942.
- Deso A. Weiss, M.D., of New York City, contributed his scheme of the mutational disturbances of the voice from the proceedings of the VIII International Speech and Voice Therapy Conference, Amsterdam, 1950.

♦ G. Panconcelli-Calzia, M.D., of Hamburg, Germany, put at my disposal a copy of his otherwise unobtainable book, *Historical Data on Phonetics.*

To these men, I wish to extend my most sincere thanks for a co-operation that was given in the spirit of the brotherhood of science.

After this book appeared for the first time, it enjoyed a wide acceptance for a number of years until it finally went out of print. The many requests for the book I received after that time from all kinds of professionals dealing with the speaking and singing voice could only be answered by referral to the public and academic libraries.

Thus, I appreciate the offer by College-Hill Press to publish this new and revised edition of the book. Mr. Linton M. Vandiver, Director of College-Hill Press, and Professor William H. Perkins of the University of Southern California have helped greatly to make this new edition possible. I hope it will be useful to a new generation of artist and professional users of the voice.

F.B.

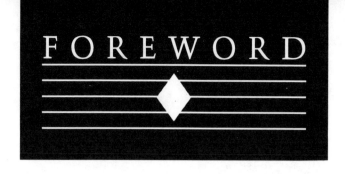

FOREWORD

*T*hese words about the distinguished laryngologist Dr. Friedrich S. Brodnitz may not be so much a foreword as an open love letter.

"Dr. Fritz," as I dubbed him affectionately, is more than a superb physician of exceptional expertise; he is a musicologist as well. Since 1961, the year of my Metropolitan Opera debut, he has been my doctor, vocal confidant, and friend. I have visited his office often without reason for an appointment, just for a laugh or two after an examination, to hear him tell me I have a bit of talent, and wish me "good luck." He lifts my morale for my next performance to the skies.

Dr. Fritz's book, *Keep Your Voice Healthy*, has been a vocal Bible for me. It contains knowledge of varying degrees and outlooks on the human voice and has heightened my understanding of my vocal organs: how to use them intelligently, their functions and production, and how to keep them healthy and sound. These rules and personal guidance from him have contributed in positive ways to my vocal longevity and health.

He is always frank, firm, critical, and objective (whether I like it or not). I am the proud possessor of a file of letters written by him after each of my performances he has attended. In these cherished letters he is not so much critical as affectionate and clearly states his pride in me and his personal enjoyment of my singing. These words I read quite often as they are a source of inspiration for me. He is one who respects and admires both my accomplishments as an opera singer and a recitalist and understands my desire to be artistically flexible.

At this stage of my life and career, I have begun to share my experiences with others, and I recommend *Keep Your Voice Healthy* as a guidepost for all singers, as well as for myself.

My heartfelt gratitude to Dr. Fritz for such tender loving care these many years, and a warm salute to him with deep admiration and respect.

Leontyne Price
New York City
April 21, 1987

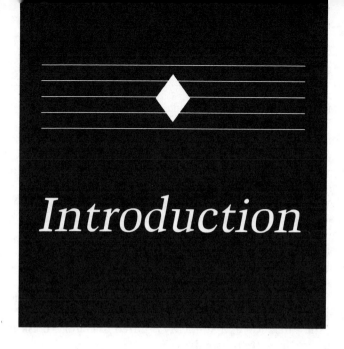

Introduction

*I*n the autumn of 1854, on one of those exquisite sunny days when Paris is at its best, a man stood in the courtyard of the Palais Royal in the midst of the stream of people who used this passage before the great boulevards were created in the reign of Napoleon III.

The man paid no attention to the palace which had seen Richelieu, the Revolution, the Empire and now the Orleans. He had no eye for the elegant stores, the coffeehouses with their little tables, and the crowd of busy Parisians, idle do-nothings, admiring strangers. He stood there in the midst of the jostling crowd with the expression of a man who has suddenly been hit by an idea.

Manuel Garcia, the most famous singing teacher of his time, then in his fiftieth year, had never been satisfied to give lessons to young artists. He had known the musical world from childhood on. The son of a great singer of Spanish birth and international reputation, he had seen the backstages of all Europe. In 1828 he even accompanied his father to New York where they presented the first stage performance of an opera in this city with *Figaro* while Mozart's librettist Lorenzo da Ponte sat in the audience.

Shortly afterward he lost his voice, which kept him from further public appearances. But out of this crisis came the determination to learn more about the human voice. Within a few years he became one of Europe's best known teachers, first in Paris and later in London, to whom students of all countries flocked. He studied all available books on anatomy and function of the vocal organs. He took part in anatomy classes, dissecting human and animal bodies until he knew more about the voice box than most doctors.

However, all this research did not satisfy him. Dead organs cannot answer questions about their function in life. Nobody had yet *seen* the human vocal cords in action, in speaking and singing. While the professionals did not pay much attention, this medical amateur had racked his brain to find the solution to the problem of making voice visible.

As it so often happens in medicine, the determined outsider had the imagination and the good luck to have the creative idea. While he stood in the Palais Royal it suddenly occured to Garcia to ask himself, *Why not try it with mirrors?*

He rushed to the store of Charriere, a maker of medical instruments, and found there a small dental mirror, left over as a failure from an exhibition in London. He bought the mirror for six francs and went back to his room to start his experiment without delay. Standing near the window he flashed the sunlight into his mouth with a large hand mirror while he introduced the small dental mirror deep into his throat with the other hand.

With a stroke of good luck, on the first attempt he chose the right angle for both mirrors and suddenly saw his own vocal folds, reflected first in the dental and from there in the large mirror.

As he described it later to his pupil Sterling MacKinlay: "There before my very eyes appeared the glottis (the space between the vocal cords) wide open ... So astounded was I that I sank back into my chair and for several minutes remained there without moving — aghast, dumbfounded. I was the first human being to see the larynx of a living man and that man was myself. Slowly I recovered from the shock and rose again to my feet. Once more I placed the dentist's mirror in the correct position, then with the larger mirror directed the ray of sunlight into the mouth ... Again the vocal cords made their appearance in the little circle of glass.

"Next I experimented in emitting various single notes, an upward scale, a downward one, an arpeggio, the registers. Then a laugh, a cry, all sorts of queer sounds, animal imitations, whatever came into my head. On and on I went, almost like a madman, until the voice was so completely tired that I had to remain silent for a long, long time."

*I*n telling you the events of this existing hour in some detail I have been guided by this reason:

The invention of the laryngeal mirror by Manuel Garcia marks the birth hour of the science of the human voice. When Garcia died in 1906, one hundred and one years old, doctors, scientists, singing teachers around the world united in a tribute to man who had given them the tool for countless new studies, for diagnosing and treating diseases of the larynx.

True, from time of antiquity on, men have tried to understand the miracle of the human voice. And after Garcia, generations of workers have labored to compile a vast literature on vocal problems. But that does not diminish the importance of the man who, in the true sense of the word, threw light into a hidden part of the human body and taught us to understand by seeing what makes us speak and sing.

There is another, and more personal, reason which makes it, in my opinion, so appropriate to begin this book with Manuel Garcia. In all his years of teaching Garcia fought for the idea that the professional user of the voice should know something about the nature and function of this instrument. In later years, this conviction even put Garcia in the paradoxical position of arguing with one of the greatest throat specialists of his time about the value of scientific knowledge for the artist and professional who lives by his voice. When Sir Morel Mackenzie expressed his doubts about the benefit a voice student could derive in his practical handling of the voice from a study of structure and function of the vocal organs, Garcia replied, "I still believe that some exact scientific notions on the formation and the action of the vocal organs would be more useful than hurtful to the rising singer."

This, then, is the basic conviction of this book, which is addressed not only to singers but to everybody who needs to use his or her voice for success. Your voice is a tool. Much more depends on the quality, the character, the handling of your voice than most people realize. People in all walks of life are hired because of the attractiveness or persuasiveness of their voices. You close a deal, you acquit a defendant as a juror, you vote for a politician, you follow your conscience after a sermon, you even marry because a voice has captivated you with just the right degree of genuine conviction, of true pathos or cool explanation, of moral zeal, or tender affection.

You influence people as often with your voice as they impress you with theirs. And you have only to remember your last case of laryngitis to understand what a handicap even a temporary impairment of your voice means in every moment of the day.

Knowledge is necessary to understand the functions of our voice, to guard its health, and to handle any danger that threatens to destroy it. This book was written bècause, as a rule, nobody told us anything about the most widely used of all instruments.

To illustrate the degree of uncertainty about the most basic facts that is common even in highly trained vocal performers, I should like to tell you about an experience which dramatically illustrates the need for better information. Years ago, a singer with considerable experience said during an examination, "Doctor, for a long time I have meant to ask somebody who knows, are the vocal cords suspended vertically or horizontally?" Before answering him I tried to find out what his conception of voice production was. It turned out that he had some vague notions about vertically placed bands, exposed to the airstream in the windpipe and made to sing in some miraculous way.

I still refused to believe that this experience could be generalized and began to ask singers, actors, teachers, and ministers the same question. I quickly realized that the right answer — that the cords are horizontally suspended — was given only by a few, and then mostly by good luck. When finally a well-known singing teacher confessed with considerable embarrassment that he knew next to nothing about the structure and function of the vocal organs, it became clear that something was wrong with the training of people who use the speaking or singing voice in their work.

Modern education has abolished the authoritarian approach of bygone days. We prefer the student who does not just imitate the teacher but asks questions, demands explanations, understands thoroughly before he accepts offered knowledge. But singers and other professionals of the voice are often still trained like seals who learn by constant obedient repetition of motions — praised when successful, scolded when not responsive, but never dignified with an explanation. They are taught the technique of free and impressive speech but they learn little about the nature and the care of their voice.

In many lectures to groups of students in music schools and seminars, in courses for adults of all walks of life, I always found great eagerness to acquire a basic knowledge in this neglected field.

Some teachers were enthusiastic, others objected. They felt that speaking and singing is a body function which should be instinctive. They believed that too much knowledge might upset the balance of this instinctive function. They even were afraid that by lifting the vocal process into the light of consciousness the singer or speaker could develop new fears and apprehensions in addition to the many that already upset him.

With Manuel Garcia, I refuse to believe that knowledge will hurt. If you ever saw the now classic film of Walt Disney's *Snow White,* you will remember the scene when Snow White, on her flight from the witch through the dark woods, finally collapses in a clearing with a circle of burning eyes surrounding her. At that moment the sun rises, revealing harmless rabbits where we expected to encounter wild and dangerous animals.

Using the vocal organs, which are hidden away in the dark recesses of our body, we are too easily the prey of the fears and anxieties that obscurity breeds. Not all wild animals can be turned into bunnies. Some dangers to the voice, as we shall see, are quite real. But the bright sunlight of knowledge will help us to separate real dangers from imagined ones, to interpet correctly sensations of all kinds in our vocal organs, to understand the mechanics of proper function and the consequences of abuse, to prevent damage, and to cooperate sensibly when help is needed.

This book is not addressed to singers alone, although we shall discuss their problems at length. Artistic singing is the highest and most specialized form of a body function which we all use in countless pursuits of life. Voice is as important to the salesperson, to the teacher, and to the courtroom lawyer as it is to the singer.

Many books have been written on improvement of elocution, speechmaking, singing techniques, enrichment of vocabulary, and polishing of speaking style. But there still is a need for a book that gives everyone who is interested in the human voice knowledge about the function and care of our vocal organs. A book alone is not a substitute for proper professional care when needed, but a book can be a guide to understanding prevention, causes, mechanisms, and treatment of voice disorders.

Voice disturbances are experienced in all walks of life. Anybody with experience in treating voice patients can easily draw up a long list of typical situations. Most of these troubles are preventable and can be avoided by better knowledge of the proper use and care of the voice and of the sources of help.

Medical terms are, to a certain extent, unavoidable. They will be explained when first used. If, later, you find that the meaning of a term has slipped your memory, the index will guide you back to the first definition.

In starting you on this conducted tour, I like to think of you as one of the students with whom I have discussed problems of the human voice in lectures and courses, and from whom came the first encouragement to write down what I tried to teach. I hope that this book will give you the information you wanted when you decided to read it.

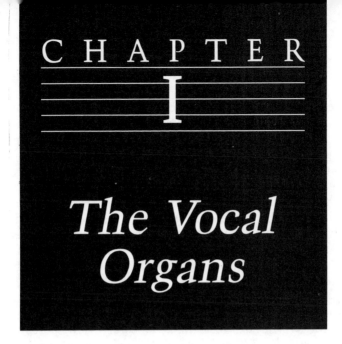

CHAPTER
I

The Vocal Organs

Any discussion of a medical subject begins with a description of the body structures involved. As long as the knowledge of the human body was limited to the visible exterior, medicine remained a mixture of superstitions, speculative theories, witchcraft, and magic traditions. Anatomy, the science of the normal human body, gained by dissection and study of organs and structures, opened the way to a real understanding of body functions and to a scientific approach to the treatment of disease.

The study of medicine begins with an intensive course in human anatomy. The physician returns constantly to anatomy books for revival and improvement of anatomical understanding. The nonprofessional cannot acquire real insight into the workings of any part of the body without the possession of a few fundamental facts about anatomy.

This poses a problem for the writer of medical books for nonprofessionals. Anatomy is a dry subject and a poor start for a book that tries to encourage the reader by attractive presentation of interesting material. The medical writer is not in the happy position of the novelist who begins with a dramatic scene and then proceeds to build up the necessary background of his story by flashbacks.

Medicine speaks a language of its own using a multitude of names and terms, describing structures, organs, functions, disturbances, and a certain minimum of "basic" language will be indispensable. Therefore, I ask your forbearance for a few pages of anatomical information about our vocal organs. I shall make it as brief as possible, avoiding the medical lingo wherever feasible.

In this connection another difficulty arises. Some parts of the body, although hidden from sight, are known to everybody, like the heart, the lungs, the stomach. For them, words exist in every language and no medical names need to be used to discuss them. Others are more or less unknown outside of the medical profession, yet fulfill important functions. Did you know, for instance, that you have a talus? Most probably not, although it is an important bone of your foot.

The vocal organs occupy a kind of linguistic middle ground. We all know — and can name them in plain English — that we have a nose, throat, voice box, vocal folds, or cords, windpipe, lungs. The diaphragm and the sinuses have kept their medical names in English, French, Italian, and the terms have become part of everyday language. But if we proceed to the inner parts of the nose or the voice box we have to use medical terms.

---

*T*he most important single feature about the vocal organs is the curious fact that none of them was originally designed by creation for the production of speech and voice. All animal life depends on a constant supply of oxygen. Fishes get it by straining oxygen from the water through the gills. Millions of years back in the course of evolution, animals began to leave water, and amphibians and mammals made their appearance. To get oxygen from air they developed lungs, connected with the outside by pipe lines from openings in the head. Noses owe their formation to the necessity of securing the vital transport of air to the lungs while the mouth is filled with food to be chewed. Even the voice box did not come into being for the production of voice, which is a rather late achievement of the higher mammals. It began as a safety valve to protect the lungs of amphibians while submerged against the choking penetration of water.

Respiration, the exchange of air between the outside and the lungs, is the primary purpose of all vocal organs — with the exception of the mouth which is part of the intake part of the digestive system too. Voice and speech have been superimposed on the organs of respiration as a kind of glorious afterthought of nature. The lungs, in addition to their function as receivers of oxygen, became bellows which blow air against the vocal folds. The folds were transformed into a musical instrument. The throat, mouth, and nose became resonating chambers to step up the volume of sound and modify voice into the richness of the spoken word.

Since these two functions — respiration and voice — are so intimately connected, the logical way to explain the anatomy of the vocal organs to you is by tracing the course of air through the *respiratory tract*. This term describes all of the structures which form the pathway of inhaled air: the nose, throat, voice box, windpipe, bronchi, lungs.

Air can enter the body in two ways, through the nose or through the mouth. If we breath quietly — for instance, sitting down and reading this book — we keep our mouth closed and inhale through the nose. The air enters the nose by way of the nostrils and travels through the nose to reach the throat. If you look at Figure I-1, which shows a cross-section through the head near the mid-line, you will be surprised by the size of the nose. You will notice that most of it is buried inside the head, and that what we commonly call our nose is just a projecting roof over the entrance to it. The nose is divided into two cavities, separated by a partition, the *nasal septum*, the *anterior* (front) rim of which you can feel between your nostrils.

The nasal septum lies in the *medial* plane of the head, and the two nasal cavities are *lateral* (on either side) of it. Anything near to an imaginary vertical plane through the middle of the body is called medial, while points farther away from it are described as lateral. The ears, for instance, are lateral of the face, the nose medial of the eyes, the nostrils are the anterior openings of the nose through which the air travels posteriorly (back) until it reaches the throat. The cross-section of the head in Figure I-1 was done slightly lateral of the midline. What you see is the outer or lateral wall of the nose, and you may be impressed or confused by the complexity of the structures. Actually, it is very simple. It is just the old engineering principle — used, for instance, in radiators and the brain — of providing maximum surface in a cramped space by folding.

You will notice three crests, projecting like the blunt edges of a clam shell. They are the *turbinates* — the Latin word for shell — decreasing in size from the bottom to the top. The recesses under the turbinates are called *meatuses*. The middle meatus — under the middle turbinate — is a strategic spot because most of the sinuses drain there into the nose. The nasal *sinuses* are bony cavities which are connected by openings with the nasal cavities. We have four pairs of them. The largest one, the *maxillary sinus* or antrum, occupies the region of the cheek, above the upper teeth and the palate and below

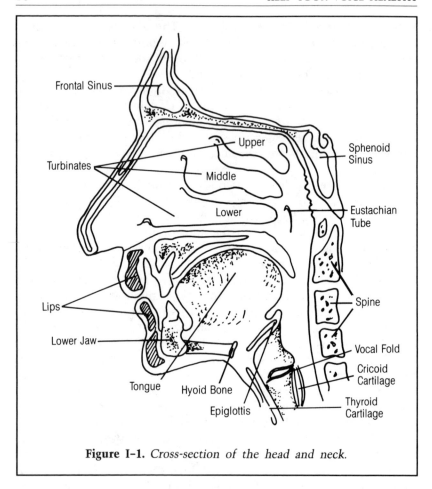

Figure I-1. *Cross-section of the head and neck.*

the eyes. The *frontal sinuses* are in the forehead, above the eyes, and are separated from each other by a thin bony partition. Between the maxillary and frontal sinuses lies a group of small cells — near the inner angle of the eyes — called *ethmoid cells*. Finally a pair of sinuses — called *sphenoids* — is buried deep in the skull, above and behind the roof of the nose.

On the cross-section of Figure I-1 you see the frontal and sphenoid sinuses, while the maxillary sinus and the ethmoid cells are hidden behind the lateral wall of the nose.

As everybody knows, the sinuses can cause a lot of trouble, although it is not yet entirely clear what their function is. Even their role as resonating chambers for the voice is extremely doubtful. The openings of the sinuses into the nasal cavities are hidden in deep recesses and are too small to permit effective passage of sound waves into the sinuses. Even filling one or more of the larger sinuses with pus or polyps changes the sound of the voice surprisingly little.

All structures of the nose, sinuses, and the whole respiratory tract down to the bronchi are lined by *mucous membranes.* As the name implies, they are constantly covered by a thin layer of mucus or phlegm produced by countless tiny glands. This blanket of mucus is kept on the move by the action of microscopically small hair-like projections of the cells of the surface, called *cilia.* In the nose, their movement is directed toward the rear — the throat; in the windpipe and bronchi, their movement is directed upward toward the throat.

Since the mucus not only lubricates all surfaces of the respiratory tract but also catches dust, dirt, and germs from the air, the ciliary action becomes part of the important self-cleaning mechanism which protects the health of the vocal folds, bronchi, and lungs. Caught on the mucous membranes, impurities of the air we inhale travel slowly to the rear of the nose into the throat where they are disposed of into the stomach by swallowing to be destroyed there by the acid of the digestive fluids. If the membranes have to work overtime, as they often do in polluted city air, we notice the appearance of mucus in our throat and call it *postnasal drip.* This is a nuisance but actually a sign that our nose is doing its job — guarding the health of the respiratory organs.

The mouth and the throat are moistened by *saliva,* the product of large glands in the cheeks (*parotid glands*) and in the floor of the mouth (*submaxillary* and *sublingual glands*). When we eat, the mechanical effect of chewing stimulates and increases flow of saliva. In addition, purely nervous impulses control the production of saliva and the action of the mucous glands. The sight of appetizing food, even the thought of it, can make our mouths water.

On the other hand, apprehension and anxiety inhibit the glands. The result is the dry mouth, tongue, and throat, a well-known experience with public speakers, actors, and singers before an appearance. When the first applause has restored the confidence, opposing impulses bring the normal flow of saliva and mucous back within a few minutes.

We all know the nose as the seat of the sense of smell, but even more important is its function as a magnificent air-conditioning unit of great simplicitity. In the very short time it takes for the air to travel from the nostrils to the throat, it is warmed to body temperature, humidified to a level of comfort for the mucous membranes, and cleaned. The folded surface of the lateral wall of the nose provides maximum contact with the air which is further increased by the curved pathway the air takes — up to the roof of the nasal cavity and down to the throat.

The size of the turbinates can be increased by filling their vessels with blood, adapting the nose to changes of temperature and dryness and following all kinds of nervous and even emotional impulses. We shall encounter this important fact frequently later on.

I have to tell you much less about the mouth because there you are on familiar ground. Let me just mention a few facts that have a bearing on voice and speech. The *tongue* is a much larger organ than we usually assume. Sticking out your tongue as widely as possible brings only the anterior part of it into the open. As you see in Figure I-1, the tongue forms a large muscular mass of crisscrossing muscle fibers which provide extraordinary flexibility and motility.

The *soft palate* with the attachment of the uvula serves as a curtain which can be raised or lowered by muscular action. When we breathe through the nose, it hangs down in relaxation and permits the passage of air into the throat. When we swallow, it is raised against the throat, thereby sealing off the nasal cavity against the penetration of food. The strong muscles of the throat do the rest, and the food is pressed downward into the gullet or *esophagus.*

I have to mention one more set of structures in the mouth that take no part in eating, breathing, or speaking but are important to health because of their nuisance value: tonsils and adenoids. Together they form a ring of so-called lymphatic tissue around the throat. The *adenoids,* as you can see in Figure I-2, form a small cushion at the roof of the throat behind the soft palate. Normally, they are present in childhood and disappear near puberty. If enlarged they block the passage of air from the nose leaving the mouth as the only free avenue. The *tonsils,* the best-known structures of the group, lie on both sides of the tongue between folds of mucous membrane in which muscles run up to the soft palate. Similar tissue is found at the base of the tongue, arranged in two small lumps that meet in the mid-line. If infected, it can form larger masses which are called *lingual tonsils* (*lingua* being the Latin name of the tongue and the root of the adjective *linguistic*). Such large lingual tonsils can form, as we shall see, a bottleneck which prevents the free development of the voice.

Behind the wall of the throat run a number of strong muscles. Aside from their action in swallowing they are able to change the form of the throat and thus modify the sound of the voice.

As you might remember, I meant to trace the pathway of air on its downward course. Leaving nose, mouth, and throat, air now reaches the point where respiratory tract and digestive system part ways. Swallowing food enters the esophagus en route to the stomach, while air passes through the voice box into the windpipe, or *trachea.*

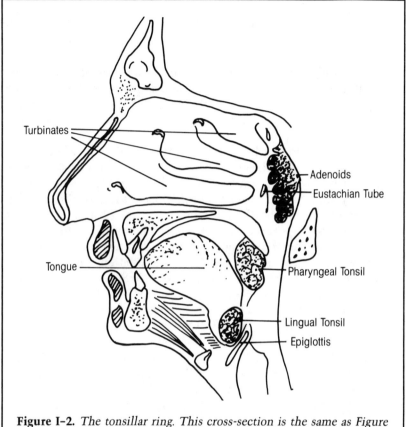

Figure I-2. *The tonsillar ring. This cross-section is the same as Figure I-1 except that the tongue has been pushed aside to make the adenoids and pharyngeal and lingual tonsils visible.*

Now we are in the chest. The air gets there through a system of pipelines, formed by division and subdivision of the windpipe. First, behind the breastbone, the trachea divides into two main *bronchi,* or bronchial tubes, one for each lung. Each main bronchus sends smaller bronchi to the lobes of the lungs, three on the right side and two on the left. Inside the lobes the bronchi become more numerous and smaller. The smallest ones are called *bronchioles* and lead the air to the air spaces of the lungs.

The whole system has been compared to a tree. But the bronchial tree is inverted. The windpipe, the trunk, is above the branches of the bronchi and bronchioles which hang down. To keep the windpipe and the bronchi from collapsing when air is sucked into the lungs, the walls of these pipelines are fortified by rings of elastic cartilage.

The lungs fill the whole chest with the exception of a space in the middle where we find the heart, the esophagus, large blood vessels, and nerves. The chest itself is a cage formed by the ribs, the spine, and the breastbone.

Lungs and heart both rest on the *diaphragm,* which got its name from the Greek word for partition. The diaphragm separates the cavities of the chest and abdomen. Since we shall have to talk a great deal about the function of the diaphragm I had better describe it to you in more detail.

The diaphragm is a large muscle. Almost all other muscles connect two points of the skeleton. By their contraction they shorten the distance between these points thereby changing the position of the bones they are attached to. The muscle fibers of the diaphragm originate from the lower ribs, the breastbone, and the spine, and converge like the spokes of a wheel at the center, which consists of tough tendinous tissues. In the relaxed position the diaphragm is dome-shaped. When the muscle fibers contract, the dome is flattened and the center moves *down.* Keep this fact in mind. We shall need it in the next chapter when we discuss the mechanism of breathing.

The lungs are covered by a protective layer of fibrous tissue, the *pleura.* A second sheet of pleura lines the inside of the chest. Both layers are connected and form the pleural sack, which contains a lubricating substance to facilite the movements of the lungs. There is no air in the pleural sack, which acts like a large suction cup that fixes the surface of the lungs to the chest wall. When the chest expands — by the elevation of the ribs — the lungs are unfolded and filled with air.

The cage of the chest is formed by the twelve pairs of ribs. They are flat bones, bent in a curvature and relatively thin, which exposes them to fractures when a severe force hits the chest. They are connected in the rear to the bones of the spine by joints with limited freedom of motion. The first seven ribs are attached to the breastbone, the next three to the higher ribs by bands of elastic cartilage which gives the chest a springy motility. The two lowest ribs are short and do not reach the breastbone. They do not take part in the movements of the chest.

Muscles between the ribs and others that are attached to the outside of the chest move the ribs up and down. The joints in the rear give leverage to the ribs which can be raised to a more horizontal position. This leads to a deepening of the chest and — in the lower half — to a sideward expansion. In this position, which is fullest in the extreme of deep inspiration, the chest has reached its greatest capacity. Moving the ribs downward contracts the chest in all dimensions, thus squeezing the air out of the lungs. We shall discuss the mechanism in more detail in the next chapter.

Leaving the air spaces of the lungs on expiration, the air passes through the bronchioles, smaller and larger bronchi, and finally the windpipe until it reaches the voice box, which we have, so far, neglected.

By now, we had better give the voice box its proper name, the *larynx*. All the medical terms for the voice box and its details are of Greek origin, proof of the interest this organ has attracted since the times of antiquity. The Greek physician Galen, who lived in the second century, described and named the larger cartilages of the larynx. The first drawings of the cartilages, the vocal folds, and the whole larynx in profile were made in 1490 by Leonardo da Vinci whose studies of the vocal organs Dr. Panconcelli-Calzia has compiled and reproduced in a beautiful volume. In the sixteenth century, Vesalius of Padua made complete dissections of the larynx that are hardly surpassed today in accuracy and detail.

The first important fact that all anatomists have noticed about the larynx is the ingenious method of suspension, which anticipated the use of springs. Above, from the jaw and base of the skull, and below, from breastbone and collarbone, muscles reach out to provide elastic suspension for the larynx and the windpipe on the top of which the voice box rides. This arrangement permits not only free movement of the larynx with the head and neck but also gives protection to the larynx from the impact of any force that hits the neck.

Above the larynx, the muscles that hold it are stabilized by the insertion of a thin bone shaped like a horseshoe (with the prongs pointing to the rear in a horizontal plane). You can feel this *hyoid bone* if you take the region slightly above your voice box between your thumb and index finger.

Added protection is given to the voice box by the fact that it is made up of highly elastic cartilage. A fracture of the larynx is a severe and sometimes fatal accident, but the free suspension and elasticity of this organ make fracture a rather rare event.

The larynx consists of nine cartilages, of which I intend to bother you with only five. The remaining four are tiny, unimportant, and belong to the large group of insignificant detail that haunts the nights of medical students before anatomy tests.

One cartilage belongs to the tongue almost as much as to the larynx. It is called *epiglottis,* and has the shape of a teaspoon with the handle sawed off (Figure I-3). You find it on the cross section of Figure I-1 too, if you look at the base of the tongue. When we swallow, the

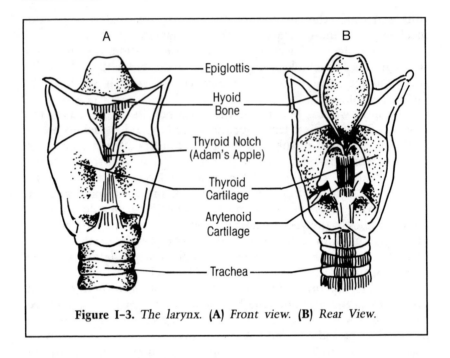

Figure I-3. *The larynx.* **(A)** *Front view.* **(B)** *Rear View.*

epiglottis tilts backward until it lies like a lid over the entrance of the larynx. Food then glides over it into the esophagus.

The "box" of the larynx is made up of two larger cartilages. The bigger one of the two consists of two wings which meet in front at a steep angle. Looking like an antique soldier's shield, it carries the Greek name for "shield-like" *thyroid* cartilage. At the upper limit of the juncture of the two shields, a deep notch can be felt with the finger. This is the most prominent part of the larynx, commonly known as the Adam's apple. In front of the lower part of the cartilage lies the important thyroid gland, which you might have heard mentioned in connection with glandular disturbances.

The wings, as they are called, do not join in the rear, thus leaving open space where no special protection is needed and where the esophagus begins behind the larynx. From the free ends of the wings two pairs of horns stick out. The inner horns connect with the hyoid bone through a band, the lower ones form a joint with the second large cartilage.

This one looks like a signet ring, with the stone facing the rear. Galen used the Greek word for ring and called it *cricoid* cartilage. It sits on top of the windpipe and connects with the thyroid cartilage by the joint I just mentioned. This makes a tilting motion of the thyroid against the cricoid cartilage possible which, as we shall see, is of importance in varying the tension of the vocal cords.

In the rear of the cricoid, on the upper rim of the "signet stone," ride two small cartilages in the shape of a pyramid with a triangular base and a tip that is slightly bent. This gives them the appearance of a pitcher and bestowed on them the tongue-twisting name of *arytenoid* cartilages. (Again I apologize in the name of the medical profession for all these unwieldly terms. They are hundreds of years old and must have given the same frustration you probably feel to countless generations of students.)

The joints that connect the arytenoids with the cricoid cartilage make two kinds of movement possible. The little pyramids can approach each other or become separated, and they can turn around an axis from the tip to the middle of the base. This is of greatest importance because attached to the anterior corners of the pyramids that face each other are the *vocal folds*. All of the structures we have mentioned so far have just one purpose: to house, protect, move, and tense the vocal folds. Since in this book we shall speak about the vocal folds more than about any other organ, they deserve a special place in our description.

It is strange to see how long the function of the vocal folds was overlooked. Even Leonardo da Vinci with his incredibly sharp eyes for detail hardly marked the folds in his drawing and believed that the voice was created in the windpipe. In 1741, Antoine Ferrein in Paris was the first scientist to understand these neglected structures as vibrating strings and called them *cordes vocales*.

The vocal folds are attached in front to the inside of the thyroid cartilage where the two wings meet. This is the fixed point where the folds always touch each other. In the rear, as I just mentioned, they are connected with the anterior corner of the arytenoids. There, they can be opened and closed, lying together on closing and forming a triangular chink on opening. This space between the opening cords is called the *glottis*.

Since this is a fundamental point, I would like you to perform a simple demonstration. Stand with your feet together. They represent the vocal folds. Where the tip of your shoes are is the firm connection of the cords with the thyroid cartilage, while your heels mark the attachment of the cords to the arytenoids. Then, spread your feet at the heels, leaving the tips of your shoes together and you have the true position of the vocal folds inside the larynx: horizontal, inseparable in front, but able to spread wide in the rear.

On the view of the larynx you see in Figure I-4 the shape of the folds becomes clearer. They are not flat bands but rather heavy and triangular on cross-section. While the upper surface is flat in the

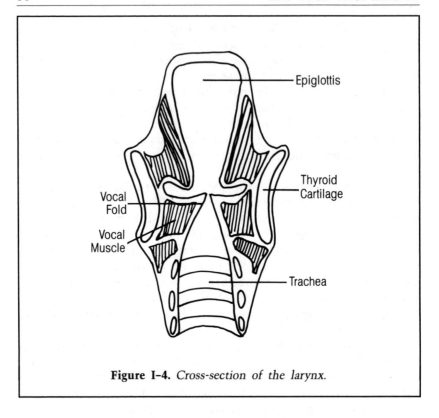

Figure I-4. *Cross-section of the larynx.*

horizontal, the lower surface slants at an angle that makes the folds thinnest at the free edges and heaviest on the outside. This slant helps to slide the air in singing and speaking against the point of contact of the folds. It is, by the way, one of the reasons why we can sing only on exhalation. Some birds have special organs, called syringes, deep down in the windpipe and can sing for minutes, on inhaling as well as on expiration.

The upper surface and the free margins which have to withstand a lot of force are covered with a tough kind of cell, somewhat similar to the top layer of our skin, while the rest of the larynx is lined with the typical mucous membrane. This accounts for the white appearance of the cords when seen from above, as on examination with the laryngeal mirror.

At this point I should like to mention that not all otherwise normal cords are white. All nuances of pinkish-gray are seen, particularly in deep voices. What is already a symptom of laryngitis for one speaker or singer may be the normal appearance for others and just the result of years of hard work like the calluses on the hands of a working man.

All normal cords have a smooth, glistening surface, due to a thin layer of mucus that covers them. Above the cords as you see in Figure I-4 are folds of mucous membrane, called the *false cords* or *false folds*. They have no special significance under normal conditions.

It remains only to tell you something about the muscles which move and tense the vocal folds. There is not much sense in bothering you with the rather complicated names of these muscles. Except for laryngologists few doctors would be able to identify the function of such tongue twisters as, for instance, the "thyroarytenoid muscle." Just look at a few drawings in Figure I-5 which explain the opening and closing of the glottis in a schematical way. You see the folds the way they are visible from above. The pyramids of the arytenoid cartilages appear as little triangles, to the anterior corner of which the posterior ends of the vocal folds are attached. The frontal ends of the folds — above in the figures — are fixed inside of the thyroid cartilages.

Two pairs of tiny muscles go from the cricoid cartilage to the outer angles of the pyramids. If the posterior pair contracts, they pull in the direction of the arrows in Figure I-5A. The pyramids are turned

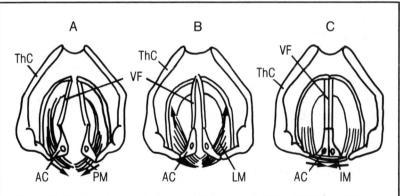

Figure I-5. *Opening and closing of the vocal folds.* (**A**) *The folds are opened by the action of the posterior mucles (PM).* (**B**) *The folds are closed by the action of the lateral muscle (LM), but a chink remains open in the posterior part.* (**C**) *The closing is completed by the action of the interarytenoid muscle (IM). ThC: thryoid cartilage; AC arytenoid cartilage; VF: vocal folds. (Pressman)*

outward and with it the vocal folds. They open wide leaving the triangular chink of the glottis between them. This is the position they assume when we breathe.

If the lateral pair of muscles contract, the arytenoids are turned inward (Figure I-5B) and the vocal folds are brought together, but in the rear an opening remains between the cartilages.

To close the last gap, muscle fibers which run from one arytenoid to the other one contract, thus pulling them together (Figure I-5C). The closure of the folds is finished. This is the position for the production of voice, but the folds cannot vibrate without being tensed. This is achieved by creating tension within and from without.

Through the whole length of each vocal fold runs a muscle. In Figure I-4 you can see it in cross-section. Contraction of this muscle makes the cords thicker, shorter, and more tense.

The tensing from without is produced by an ingenious mechanism. As you may remember, the thyroid cartilage can be tilted against the cricoid. This movement, which is achieved by another muscle, lengthens the distance between the two points of attachment of the vocal folds. Result: the cords are stretched, becoming longer, thinner, and more tense.

Both mechanisms, increase of the inner tension of the cords and stretching by outside pull, combine to produce any desired degree of tension, length, and thickness of the vocal folds. You can visualize this interplay of forces by using one of the flat rubber bands that are used to hold small parcels. If you take one loop in one hand so that two sections of the band are parallel and approximated, and pull the other end you will observe the thinning of the bands while you feel the increased inner tension of the stretched bands.

This finishes our excursion into the anatomy of the vocal organs. We can now proceed to the study of the mechanism of voice production.

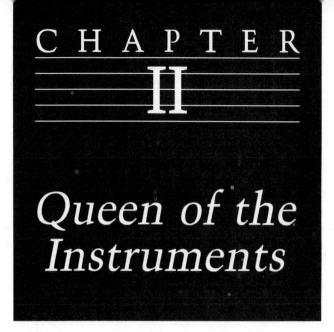

CHAPTER II

Queen of the Instruments

The stage is set for the great aria of "Leonore" in Beethoven's *Fidelio*. A stormy recitative paints the uproar of the elements with strings and woodwinds. Three horns, one after the other one, introduce a moving phrase in the radiant yet mellow harmonies of E-major.

But then, the voice emerges, the voice of a woman who trembles for her captive husband, and suddenly all the instruments of the orchestra pale beside the flexibility, the grandeur, and the richness of this singular instrument. It sings of fear, of despair, and of prayerful hope until it finally erupts into the quickened pulses of courage and determination. One cannot hear this masterpiece of musical creation interpreted by a great singer without being touched to tears.

It is not a powerful instrument, this human voice, nor a technically perfect one. A trumpet can blow louder, a violin can play faster, an oboe can spin longer melodies. Still, it is unsurpassed in expressivity, depth and soulfulness of tone, truly the queen of instruments.

The voice is not the property of the singer alone. It colors every word we say with emotional undertones, with pathos or humble resignation, with energy or deadly fear, with persuasiveness or deceit. We use this instrument daily and still know very little about it. This chapter intends to introduce you to the mechanics of the voice. We are still far away from having all the answers about the function and the acoustics of the voice. Many details are still hotly argued about. But we can, at least, explain satisfactorily the basic facts of voice production in simplified terms.

Whether we use the voice in speaking or singing, we produce — in acoustical terms — vibrations of air. Every audible sound consists of such vibrations: rhythmical ones in music, irregular ones in noise. To leave the latter out for the time being, we can say that every musical note corresponds to a rhythmical vibration of air, called *frequency*, measured in vibrations per second. From the point of origin the *waves* of sound spread in all directions, weakening in the square of distance until they die away. The greater the motion of vibrating air, the greater the *amplitude*, or intensity, of the sound.

Outside of experimental setups hardly any pure tones are produced in nature. Any sound that emanates from an instrument or from the voice consists of a basic tone, the *fundamental* tone, and a number of related *overtones* or *partials*, which are usually multiples of the basic frequency. The mixture of the fundamental with partials of varying strength accounts for the color or quality which distinguishes for our ear the same note if played by a violin or an oboe, by a flute or a clarinet, or if sung by a soprano or an alto.

Every note of our harmonic system has a certain frequency or *pitch*. The intervals we use in all kinds of musical compositions can be expressed in relations of frequencies. The higher note of an octave has twice the number of vibrations as the lower one. The major triad — the basis of our musical system — has frequency values of 4:5:6.

Instruments can be classified according to the mechanics they employ in creating vibrations of air. We can best understand the mechanism of the human voice if we compare it to the major instrumental groups of the orchestra.

Woodwinds and brass instruments are both, acoustically speaking, pipes. A column of air, enclosed in a wooden or metal pipe, is made to vibrate.

In the woodwinds, with the exception of the flute, this is achieved by the action of reeds. Flat pieces of thin slices of cane are mounted on a mouthpiece. When blown against, they begin to vibrate, opening and closing the entrance of the mouthpiece. The steady stream of air is rhythmically interrupted, and the resulting vibration of air is transmitted to the air in the wooden body of the instrument. While the clarinet employs a single reed, the oboe and the bassoon have two reeds in close contact (see Figure II-1). In the opening phase they swing away from each other, separated by the pressure of air and return again to the closed position by their elasticity. The vibration of the vocal folds has been compared to this double-reed action.

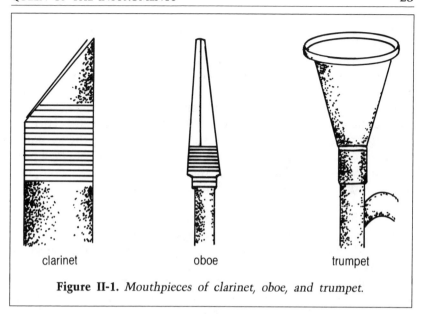

Figure II-1. *Mouthpieces of clarinet, oboe, and trumpet.*

The principle of action of the brass instruments gives an even better illustration. Here, the lips of the player are the source of air vibration. Pressed under tension into the funnel-shaped mouthpiece, they open and close to the blowing stream of air in quick succession. The tense but rounded margins of the lips act like vibrating cushions which have given to this type of instrument the acoustic name of *cushion pipes.*

The vocal folds are also cushion pipes. Closed and tensed, they resist the pressure of air in the trachea until they are blown apart. A puff of air escapes and lowers the air pressure below. The temporary decrease of pressure permits the closure of the folds by their inner tension and elasticity. This interplay of forces achieves a fast rhythmical change of opening and closing, thus transforming the steady stream of air into rhythmical vibrations. The tone is born.

In most pipe instruments the pitch of the sound they produce depends on the length of the vibrating air column. The shorter the column, the higher the pitch. Through a system of keys or valves which open holes to the escape of air, the length of the pipe can be varied and a series of different tones produced.

The human voice employs a different principle to achieve changes in pitch: the increase or decrease of the tension of the vocal folds. We find the same principle used in all string instruments. A violin, for instance, is tuned to the desired pitch by turning the pegs which hold the strings, thereby changing the tension. The higher the tension the faster the vibrations and the higher the produced note. The fingering in playing the string instruments has the same effect. Shortening the vibrating part of the string increases the tension and raises the pitch.

Increase or decrease of the tension of the vocal folds is achieved by the muscular mechanism we discussed in the last chapter. If we want to sing a higher note after a lower one, we increase the tension of the folds and thus make them vibrate at a faster rate. If you tie a piece of string at one end and pull on the other end, you can produce a whole series of sounds by plucking the string at different degrees of tension.

The intensity, or loudness, of a given note depends on the degree of air pressure from below. The harder we blow against the folds, the wider the vibrating excursions of the folds and the louder the sound our voice produces.

Actually, an increase in air pressure raises the pitch to a certain degree, but a fine adjustment of the tensing muscles of the folds compensates for this effect. For our purposes, we can stick to our definition: increased tension of the folds raises the pitch, increased pressure of air fortifies the intensity of the sound.

The frequency of a given tone determines the speed with which the folds vibrate. The deepest notes of a basso require around 60 vibrations of the folds per second. For the a¹ on the second space of our usual treble clef — the so-called chamber A — 440 vibrations are necessary. But for the high c³ of a soprano the vocal folds have to open and close at the incredible speed of 1,046 vibrations per second.

Observations with the high-speed camera — which we shall discuss in Chapter XIII — have taught us a great deal about the vibrations of the folds. They do not close or open in a straight line but in a rather undulating fashion. In slow motion it looks like a blanket being shaken in waves. This means that at no time in singing is the whole length of the folds completely closed.

There exists a fundamental difference in the type of vibration at low and high tones. In producing low notes, the folds swing wide with a movement that envelops the whole mass of the folds. The higher the note, the more limited the vibration to the free borders of the folds becomes. Finally, in the highest notes the folds remain in close contact in the posterior part, leaving only the anterior half or third free to vibrate. At this stage the folds are tense, show no motion in the rear, and vibrate in the frontal part only at the sharpened inner margins.

For a better visualization of the motion of the folds you should now turn to Figures II-2 through II-6, which show a number of photographs taken under different conditions of vocal use.

Figure II-2 shows a set of photographs of the folds during one full cycle of opening and closing in singing. They are single exposures which were taken out of a film that was obtained with a high-speed camera. Since during this shot the singer produced a note of about 260 vibrations, the set of the six photographs covers the time of 1/260 second.

Figure II-3 (from the same film) shows the folds of a baritone singing three different notes. The second one is an octave higher than the first, the third one is one-fifth higher than the second. The higher the note, the thinner and longer the folds become by stretching.

Figure II-4 shows the position of the folds in singing high notes. At the beginning of the head register (A), the folds are stretched but still vibrate at full length. Higher up (B), the folds are approximated (damped) at the posterior half, leaving the anterior half free to vibrate. In falsetto (C), the folds are damped in the two posterior thirds; only a small triangular chink is open in the anterior third where the sharpened margins vibrate.

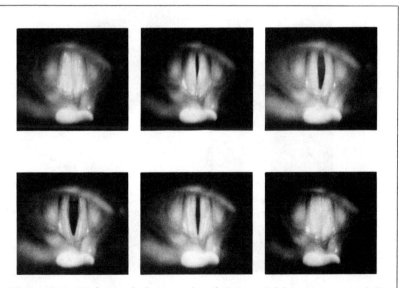

Figure II-2. *High-speed photographs of the vocal folds during one full cycle of opening and closing. (Courtesy of Bell Telephone Laboratories)*

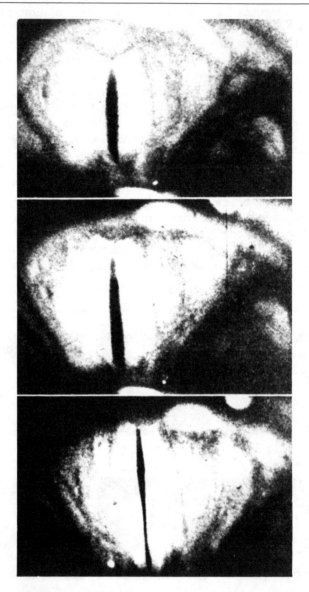

Figure II-3. *Elongation of the true vocal folds with pitch. From top to bottom, the photographs represent three stages in the gradual transition from singing a lower tone (about 120 Hz) to a higher tone (about 300 Hz). (Courtesy of Bell Telephone Laboratories.)*

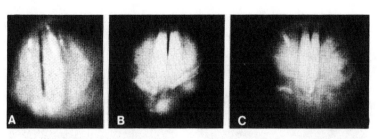

Figure II-4. *Position of the vocal folds while singing progressively higher notes.* **(A)** *The folds are stretched but still vibrate along their full length.* **(B)** *The folds are approximated at the posterior half, leaving the anterior half free to vibrate.* **(C)** *The folds are approximated in the two posterior thirds, with only a small triangular chink open in the anterior third. (Courtesy of Bell Telephone Laboratories.)*

Figure II-5 illustrates the different degrees of fold opening in breathing, from quiet respiration (A), to moderate work (B), such as walking on the street, and to breathing in extreme exertion (C) with wide open folds, between which the upper rings of the windpipe can be seen.

I would like to mention here the position of the folds in *whispering* because of its great practical importance. Figure II-6 shows the folds in both toneless whispering (A) and in the more forceful "stage" whisper (B). You can see that in both instances the folds are approaching each other, in the forceful whisper to the point of contact. In both conditions they vibrate. Therefore, whispering is *no* rest for the vocal folds. If vocal rest is needed, whispering as well as speaking should be avoided.

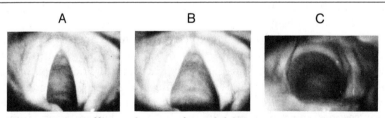

Figure II-5. *Different degrees of vocal fold opening in breathing.* **(A)** *During quiet respiration.* **(B)** *During moderate work.* **(C)** *During extreme exertion. (Courtesy of Bell Telephone Laboratories.)*

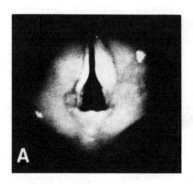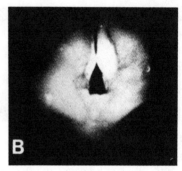

Figure II-6. *Position of the vocal folds during whispering.* **(A)** *Toneless whisper.* **(B)** *Stage whisper.*

So far, I have discussed only the vocal folds as the source of sound. If we heard only the sound the folds produce, we would perceive a weak, tinny voice, hardly audible at more than a few feet distance. The same applies to most musical instruments. The strings of a violin, for instance, would produce only a very weak sound without the help of the resonating body of the instrument. *Resonance* describes any process by which the energy of a musical sound is augmented. The weak vibrations of the strings of the violin are taken over and reinforced by the vibrations of the wooden body of the instrument which, in turn, incites the air inside the body to strong vibrations, all resulting in a tone of great intensity. The body is the resonator of the violin.

Such resonators can be selective — sharply attuned to one single frequency, such as the pipes of an organ, or they can be broad resonators which amplify a wide range of sounds. The horn of a loudspeaker, the bell of the brass instruments, and the sounding board of a piano are such broad resonators.

The resonator of the human voice is unique because its shape can be partly altered. Of the organs which enclose the air column above the vocal cords only the nose is a rigid structure. The shape of the throat and, more so, of the mouth, tongue, and lips can be changed by muscular action. As we shall see, speech is made possible by changes of the resonating cavities, and the quality of musical sound in singing can be considerably altered by conscious and subconscious modifications of the resonators.

The human resonator is predominantly the broad type. Hard and rigid resonators have a more selective effect than those with softer surfaces that give a more general reinforcement of sounds. This result is based on the filtering out of overtones by absorption, the so-called damping effect. Selective resonance produces more powerful tones, but the soft and changeable walls of the human resonator permit the production of a wide range of usable sounds.

Resonance is not limited to the air spaces above the vocal folds. To a certain extent, the air in the windpipe and bronchi takes part in the amplification of sound, particularly in the deep tones up to frequencies of 250. While speaking with our deepest voice or singing in the low range, we can feel the resonating vibrations in our chest.

At this point, I would like to say a word about vibrations as body sensations. Many speakers, when speaking forcefully, as to a large crowd, and most singers when singing loudly can feel all kinds of vibrations in the palate, the nose, the forehead, and in other places. These sensations have led many teachers to the false concept that sound could be "directed" selectively to such parts of the body. From one individual to another, the body sensations vary greatly; they have no significance for the right or wrong use of the voice and are not a key to the improvement of singing or speaking techniques.

Whether we speak or sing, we always use the vocal organs as a unit. Physicists call it a *coupled system*. That means that its sound-producing parts, the vocal folds with the air columns above and below, act together, one influencing, reinforcing, and stimulating the vibrations of the other. Any teaching theory that picks out a single sensation or movement as a guide to perfection leaves the firm basis of scientific fact.

So far, I have discussed the vocal folds, which are the source of voice sounds, and the resonating cavities, which step up the volume of sound to its full dynamic possibilities. It remains to consider the bellows which provide the air pressure and drive the vocal folds to vibration.

In the last chapter, we described the mechanism of the *chest* in *breathing*, based on the raising and lowering of the ribs. This breathing by expansion and contraction of the chest is supplemented by *abdominal breathing*. You will remember that the dome-shaped diaphragm flattens and descends on contraction during deep inspiration (Figure II-7A).

All muscles of the human body are arranged in opposing pairs. Each muscle or muscle group corresponds to another one that acts as its antagonist. For instance, if you bend your forearm, you contract the biceps muscle while its antagonist, the triceps, relaxes. This muscle, in turn, takes over if you wish to extend the arm. Then, the triceps contracts and the antagonist, the biceps, relaxes.

The antagonists of the diaphragm are the muscles which tense the abdominal wall (belly and flanks). In deep inspiration the diaphragm contracts and moves down. This exerts pressure on the organs

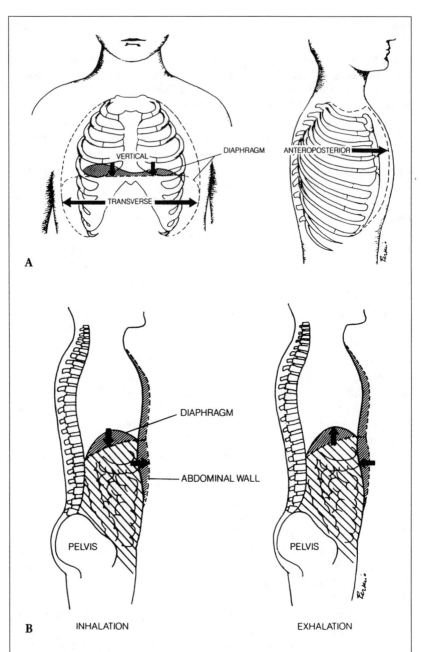

A

B   INHALATION   EXHALATION

Figure II-7. *The mechanics of breathing.* **(A)** *Chest movement.* **(B)** *Diaphragm and abdominal movement. (Adapted from Perkins, W. H., and Kent, R. D. (1986). Functional anatomy of speech, language, and hearing. San Diego: College-Hill Press.)*

which fill the abdominal cavity, the liver, stomach, intestines, and others. To escape the downward pressure from above, they begin to protrude. This is made possible by the relaxation of the abdominal muscles. The result of this mechanism is more air space in the chest because of the flattening of the diaphragm, and expansion of the belly to accommodate the protruding abdominal organs (Figure II-7 B).

Now, let us consider what happens in deep expiration, for instance, while we speak or sing. The diaphragm relaxes and the abdominal muscles contract. The abdominal organs are compressed by the contracting muscles. To escape this pressure they move inward and upward, pushing the relaxing diaphragm into the chest, thus squeezing air out of the lungs. At the end of a deep expiration, the wall of the abdomen and flanks is pulled in, and the relaxed diaphragm has risen until it has assumed its dome shape (Figure II-7B).

This interplay of forces, if done well, goes very smoothly; contraction and relaxation are perfected in slow transitions. But one fact is clear from this explanation: In abdominal inspiration, the driving force is the diaphragm, while expiration is controlled by the abdominal muscles. The term *diaphragmatical control,* which has become such a favorite with teachers of singing and speaking, is somewhat misleading. During expiration, when we create air pressure to make the vocal folds vibrate, it is the abdominal muscles that do the real work.

A smooth control of expiration depends to a certain degree on the slow relaxation of the diaphragm, but another factor prevents a conscious control of the diaphragm. Of all the muscles of the human body the diaphragm is the only one without a sense of position. Even with closed eyes we are always aware of the position of all of the parts of our body. In breathing, we can feel the action of all parts involved. We are aware of the expansion or contraction of our chest. We can feel the contraction or the bulging of our belly and our flanks. But we cannot become aware of the position of our diaphragm in breathing. For this reason, it would be better to speak of *abdominal control,* but *diaphragmatic control* has become such a favorite with the singing profession that the term will stay, regardless of the functional facts. Not much harm will be done as long as you are fully aware of the antagonistic interplay of both muscle groups.

We all use chest and abdominal breathing together. As a rule, chest breathing is more pronounced in women and abdominal breathing is more pronounced in men. The goal of proper training of the speaking and singing voice is to strengthen the less developed mechanism and to blend both into one smoothly functioning unit. There is no one prescription for ideal breathing. It is the task of a good teacher to find out which form of breathing gives the best results in an individual student.

The trouble with too many systems of vocal instruction is that they try to make everybody conform to a rigid set of motions and actions. Some of the best singers have used highly irregular positions and movements of their vocal organs. And the brilliant result that a system has achieved with one student does not prove that it will be successful with others. The best teacher is the one who is able to develop the possibilities of each student using flexible methods and techniques.

In quiet breathing, expiration takes about fifty percent more time than inspiration. This ratio is changed in speaking or singing when the expiration becomes prolonged enough to permit the speaking of an entire sentence or the singing of a complete musical phrase in one breath. Nose breathing, which permits the intake of air only at a slower rate, becomes insufficient for the needs of speedy inspiration in speaking and singing — as it does in strenuous exercise — and then we switch to mouth breathing.

The beneficial effect of nose breathing is still preserved because even the busiest speaker or singer keeps his mouth closed for the greater part of the day. Aside from the air-conditioning function of the nose, nasal breathing is of great importance to the strengthing of the voice. If you breathe first through mouth and then through the nose, you will notice the resistance that the narrower pathway of the nose offers to breathing. This helps to develop the muscles which are involved both in inspiration and expiration, particularly in younger individuals.

*N*ow, we can bring the whole picture into focus. We have discussed the mechanism of breathing which provides air pressure below the vocal folds. The folds, which are closed and tensed at the beginning of phonation, are blown apart by the mounting air pressure in the trachea and then made to vibrate by the interplay of pressure from below and the elastic resistance in the folds. The resulting vibration creates a sound which is amplified in the resonating cavities. Pitch depends on the frequency of vibration of the folds, the volume of sound depends on the pressure of air against the folds.

We still have to discuss a number of details which are important for the understanding of artistic singing, but before doing so, we should first study the mechanics of speech, the characteristics of the speaking voice, and the requirements for professional speech. The next two chapters will be used for this purpose; we will then return to the singing voice in Chapter V.

B efore we can close this chapter I have to touch on one more subject: the functions of the larynx aside from the production of voice.

I started this anatomical description with the remark that the larynx appeared first in amphibians as a safety valve against penetration of water into the newly developed lungs. With the economy that is so characteristic of the evolution in nature, this valve was maintained in the mammals but adapted to new functions, which have to do with the building up of air pressure in the chest by tight closure of the folds during expiration.

When some animals developed the ability to do heavy work with their forelimbs while squatting on their haunches, they learned how to get added strength for lifting heavy objects by suddenly closing the folds and pressing air against them. This action transforms the chest into a rigid cage, which gives the muscles of the forelimb that are attached to it greater power and a firmer grip. Humans, who transformed their forelimbs into the adaptable and versatile tools of the arms, use this technique constantly. If we want to lift a heavy crate, we first close our vocal folds tightly, build up air pressure by contraction of the chest and abdominal muscles, and then use the muscles of the arms. When the work is done we release the air with an audible rush and resume normal breathing. People who have lost the ability to close the folds or who have to wear a cannula in the trachea after an operation are severely handicapped for heavy work.

I also might mention here that this evolution process has been paid for by choking up our airways. In assuming this posture, the pathway of air in the throat has become bent at a sharp angle. When running fast, we assume instinctively the animal position of the head by thrusting our chin forward and upward, thus straightening out the throat for greater efficiency of intake of air.

Another use of the larynx as a valve is made in coughing, when we use the sudden release of pressure behind the closed folds to eject mucus from trachea in bronchi with the rush of escaping air. One more use of the pressure-valve mechanism is made in bowel movements when the compressed air in the chest forces the diaphragm down, thus providing pressure on the intestines in teamwork with the contracting abdominal muscles.

All in all, it is the story of the versatility of nature we have followed in the last two chapters. Dr. V. E. Negus, a famous English throat specialist, wrote a fascinating study of the evolutionary history of the larynx. Dissecting the larynxes of hundreds of different animals, he traced its development from a simple valve to the most magnificent musical instrument in existence. He also showed that the conditions of life, not the anatomical structures, have determined the use of the larynx for voice.

Animals living in open spaces (e.g., giraffes, antelopes) have no need for voices. Some higher animals have all of the structures of the human larynx, yet use no voice. However, in humans, greater brain power created the need for a better form of communication. The mouth, the entrance to the digestive system, became the instrument for *speech,* the finest of all human achievements. Speech is the topic of the next chapter.

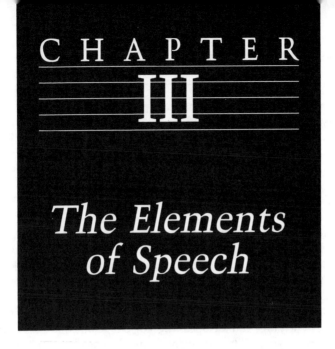

CHAPTER

III

The Elements
of Speech

*I*n a sense, our real lives as human beings begin with the
moment when the first word leaves our lips. It takes us a year
and often longer to reach this stage. The cry of our first days —
a protest against a cold and hostile new world — becomes more vari-
able and differentiated, but for months it still takes the loving
interpretation of the parents to identify the expressions of pleasure or
anger, of hunger or pain.

Slowly we begin to experiment with sounds. We go through the
"babbling" stage, producing an increasing variety of vocal combinations. We echo syllables in nonsensical repetition, we imitate
speech sounds in clumsy distortion. And finally the first word makes
its appearance. Up to that point, we have little to show that we are in
any way superior to the higher animals. We are even more helpless
and longer in need of the constant care of our mothers. The moment
that sets us really apart from all other beings is the birth of the first
word. From that hour on we belong to humanity.

We need years to complete the miracle of fully developed speech.
Our vocabulary grows from 10 to 20 words at eighteen months to 50
to 250 words at the end of the second year and 800 to 900 words at the
end of the third year. And it keeps growing through most of our life.
We learn to put words together, first in simple combinations, then in
whole sentences. From the use of words as simple labels for persons
and objects, we graduate to their higher applications: to express

desires, to describe events, to define groups and categories, to formulate abstractions and ideas.

Speech is voiced breath, modified by *articulation* (the movements which change the shape and form of the cavities above the vocal folds). The throat, the soft palate, the tongue, and the lips, singly or in groups, produce a tremendous variety of such changes which mold the airstream into the individualities of speech sounds.

The voice provides the level, the intensity, and the range of speech. The average female speaking voice is about one octave higher than the male voice. The mean fundamental frequency (pitch) of the male voice for vowels lies at about 124 vibrations per second (corresponding to the B of the musical scale). For the female voice, it lies at about 244 vibrations per second (the b of the musical scale). These values also vary with the types of voices, deep and high ones.

The average pitch level of an individual's voice can be determined by listening to his speech and comparing it with tuning forks or whistles of standard pitch. It requires a good ear and much practice.

In actual speaking we constantly deviate in small intervals — thirds or fourths — from our basic level. In addition, the voice level of our speech is raised or lowered by emotional changes. Fear, excitement, anger, joy, and many other emotions push our voice up or down, far from the level we use in contentment and equanimity.

Out of the raw materials of the voice we form, by modification of the airstream, the speech sounds that constitute the elements of the spoken word. We use a large number of them, many more than the letters of the alphabet we learned in school. To discuss the mechanics of each sound would lead us too deep into the underbrush of phonetics.

I shall confine this discussion to the general principles that rule the production of speech elements. For this purpose, I can use the well-known classification of vowels and consonants, but you have to keep in mind that I am going to describe speech sounds, not the letters of the printed or written alphabet.

The ability to voluntarily change the shape of the lips and mouth is a rather late achievement in evolution. Reptiles and birds have no lips and cheeks, only rigid structures of the mouth. Of the mammals, the apes have muscular mouth cavities of great pliability, but only man has learned to control them to the degree of changing the resonating qualities.

In describing vowels we are confronted with a difficulty we shall encounter frequently in this chapter: the letters of the conventional alphabet are insufficient to identify vowels and consonants clearly. In languages with phonetic spelling, like Italian, the letters A, E, I, O, U conform, to a high degree, to the actual speech sounds. The English language is blessed with a grammar of great simplicity and with a vocabulary the richness of which satisfies the scientist and the poet alike, but is cursed with an antiquated and completely erratic spelling.

The child, luckily, begins to speak long before learning to read. A small child is not bothered by the fact that in saying "father," "stranger," and "salt" three different vowel sounds are used, although the same letter of the alphabet appears in the printed word. But the adult who has lost the ability of picking up language by ear and who needs books for the learning of a new tongue finds this discrepancy between symbol and sound very confusing.

As an added complication, the English language is rich in *diphthongs,* combinations of two different succeeding vowels. Here, too, spelling gives no reliable clue.

To get some order into the great variety of vowel sounds, they have been classified according to articulatory movements into *front, middle,* and *back vowels.* According to this classification, typical front vowels are used in saying "beat," "bit," "bait," "bat," "bet;" middle vowels in "ask," "bird," "above;" back vowels in "fore," "full," "fall," "hot," "calm." Acoustically speaking, all of these sounds are mixtures of a basic frequency, the fundamental, with a number of overtones or partials, that were discussed in the last chapter.

Vowels, according to the source/filter theory of speech, are generated by vocal fold tone and then are modified by the resonance cavities of the throat, mouth, and nose. Widening or narrowing of the mouth or throat changes the resonating properties of the cavities above the vocal folds. This makes it possible to create a great variety of fundamental–partial mixtures, resulting in different vowel sounds. The overtones of vowels are mostly of the harmonic type. With modern equipment for sound analysis, up to thirty-five different overtones have been registered in a single vowel sound.

Consonants are produced by a different mechanism. The airstream is deflected, hindered, or interrupted by obstacles we put into its way. We call the places where such obstacles are created the *zones of articulation.* There are three of them. The first zone lies between the lips or between the lower lips and the upper front teeth. Consonants in this group are P, B, W, Wh, F, V, and M.

The second zone is found between the front teeth, the tip of the tongue, and the hard palate behind the teeth. In this group are T, D, Th, R, L, S, Sh, Zh, Y, and N. In the third zone are the sounds formed by the back of the tongue and the soft palate. To this group belong K, G, and Ng (as in "long").

Another classification of consonants can be gained by considering the type of obstruction they require. If a complete interruption of the airstream is needed, we call these sounds *plosives*, because the air pressure is first built up behind the obstruction and then suddenly released in a tiny explosion. B and P are formed in this manner by the lips, T and D by the tip of the tongue and the hard palate, and K and G by the back of the tongue and the soft palate.

If the airstream is not completely interrupted but forced through a narrow passage we call the resulting sounds *fricatives.* If you speak F, V, Th, S, Z, or H, you can feel and hear the air hissing through the narrow slits at the various points of formation.

Some consonants, like W, are spoken with a *gliding* movement. They are half consonant, half vowel in character.

A third classification is based on the presence or absence of vocal fold vibration. We call these consonants *voiced* or *voiceless.* If you pronounce first a P and then a B, by placing your finger at the bottom of your mouth, you can feel the vibration of the folds in the B while they are absent in the P. To the group of voiced consonants belong B, D, G, V, and Z; the voiceless ones include P, T, K, F, S, and Sh.

The *nasal* sounds are in a category by themselves. All of the speech sounds of the English language, with the exception of three, are spoken with a raised soft palate. In this position the airstream is prevented from reaching the nose and is directed into the mouth. In three speech sounds, M, N, and Ng (as in string), the palate is lowered, thus opening the door into the nose. In M the lips close the way through the mouth, N tongue and lips, and in Ng the back of the tongue and the soft palate. If you place your fingertip at the outside of the nostrils, you will feel the vibration in these nasal sounds. In French the vowels preceding nasal consonants are spoken with nasality too — one of the reasons why a good French pronunciation is so hard for English-speaking people.

So far, I have given you just the bare outline of the mechanics of speech sounds. Most likely, you are already quite bewildered by the complexity of a process that seems so simple when we use it in daily speech. Still, you can thank your lucky stars that you were born into one of the Western languages. There is no end to the variety of composite speech movements, from double stops in African languages, glottal stops in Dutch, to side-of-the-tongue sounds in Japanese. In Northern Chinese groups of speech sounds may give four different meanings if spoken with changed intonation.

If we apply our acoustical knowledge to the consonants, we find that the partials or overtones which give them their characteristic color belong — in contrast to the vowels — more to the class of noises. The fricatives, like S or F, have particularly high frequencies in their overtones.

In analyzing speech frequencies it has been found that the higher frequencies are very important for the intelligibility of speech. One can filter all the frequencies under 500 out of our speech and still obtain understandable communication, but the high frequencies cannot be eliminated without resulting in blurring. This explains the difficulties of the patient with a deafness that affects the acuity of the hearing nerve. In this type of deafness, which often occurs with aging, the high frequencies are the first ones to suffer. Although music can still be enjoyed to a certain degree, the understanding of speech deteriorates increasingly because of the loss of hearing in the high frequency zone.

All of the mechanisms we have so far discussed are part of the so-called normal voice and speech production. We say "so-called" because there is no one alive who fulfills in speech and voice all of the requirements of normal function. Even the finest singers and speakers manage, at best, to come near to what we consider perfect and, therefore, normal function.

In the field of speech sounds, many outside influences modify the mechanics of production of vowels and consonants. Regional customs in the form of dialects and local speech habits lead to omission and modulation of speech sounds or to the substitution of "normal" sounds by others. The whole melody and inflection of speech can be involved, creating new local "normalities" that would be irregular elsewhere. Think of the Southern "drawl" or the New England "twang." In the case of the latter, the characteristic voice of the Yankee is produced by a constriction of the glottis and by contraction of the lower part of the throat. You can produce the same effect by placing the flat hand against the region above the larynx and pressing hard upward and backward.

A famous example of the willful substitution of speech sounds is *ventriloquism*. This form of artificial speech has always intrigued scientists. In 1772 the French Abbé de la Chapelle wrote the first treatise on ventriloquism. His rather obscure explanations were vastly improved by T. Flatau and H. Gutzmann — two pioneers in our field — who in 1894 published the results of careful studies on ventriloquism. The ventriloquist uses the same vocal organs as we do. The biggest problem is to avoid all speech sounds of the frontal zone of articulation, since any movement of the lips would instantly destroy the illusion. The ventriloquist has to learn to use contractions of the throat and soft palate together with retraction of the base of the tongue to produce substitute speech sounds. From these maneuvers the voice of the ventriloquist acquires its typical pressed quality.

*N*ow let us return to a problem we have touched already, the relationship between speech sounds and the written or printed word.

All Western languages use systems of letters to build up words. Some languages, like Italian, nearly approach the ideal of identifying the spoken sound by a letter of the alphabet. For the student of French or German, it is more difficult to guess the correct pronunciation from the combination of letters used. But English has one of the most irregular and imprecise ways of defining the spoken word by alphabetical symbols. The discrepancy between spelling and pronouncing is very great in our language.

You have only to look at the following pairs of words to realize how often similar spelling is used for different pronunciations, or the same sound is spelled differently.

pride—birth	laugh—because	general—again
father—danger	good—moon	long—danger
reach—death	you—try	whole—white
soul—out	cow—blow	under tutor

This system — or should one rather say confusion — of spelling is one of the main reasons why so many children in the United States have difficulties in learning how to read. To coordinate a group of letters to a spoken word is easier for a child in a language with phonetic spelling.

For the purposes of speech analysis and research, a *phonetic alphabet* that uses different symbols for each speech sound would be a great help. Many such phonetic alphabets have been constructed. The best so far, and most widely accepted one, is the alphabet on which the International Phonetic Association has agreed. It uses 63 symbols for consonants and 28 for vowel sounds. At least 41 of these symbols (15 for vowels and 26 for consonants) are necessary to identify the speech sounds of American English.

Most of the larger dictionaries employ their own simplified phonetic system to indicate the pronunciation of a word, but in each the number of such "letters" is larger than the 26 of the alphabet. All phonetic alphabets have the same limitations: nobody has yet devised a system that includes all of the speech sounds used in human languages. Human speech is too rich to be fully mirrored in printed symbols. No letter can ever do justice to the countless varieties which the habits of language, country, region, and individuality impress on spoken sounds.

---

*B*efore closing this chapter a last word should be said about the *control of the speaking voice by the brain.* All of the actions and functions of our bodies can be grouped into voluntary and involuntary ones. For instance, we move arms or legs by voluntary muscular contractions, but our hearts beat rhythmically, independently of our will. The involuntary functions are under the supervision of the *autonomic nervous system,* which consists of a number of centers in the brain and a chain of nerve control points in the body. Voluntary actions are controlled by centers which are located on the surface of the two halves of the brain. The gray *cortex,* as the outer layer is called, contains the centers for body movements and sensations.

Breathing, the driving force of the vocal organs, is a mixed voluntary–involuntary function. If we sleep or, while awake, pay no attention to our breathing, it goes on quite automatically in a steady rhythm. The *respiratory center,* like the automatic steering of a modern plane, keeps the breathing going. But the pilot, the cortex, can at any time take over. We are able to breathe with voluntary control at any desirable depth, provided that we respect the oxygen needs of the body. We cannot suppress breathing beyond a relatively short period.

In ordinary speaking, we are not aware of our breathing movements but the actor is, at least when he tries to arrange a long passage in artistically satisfying breathing periods. The student of speaking or singing may begin with exercises for voluntary breathing control. The singer when studying a part uses conscious breathing. With improved technique, with greater familiarity with an aria, breathing again becomes automatic. In short, breathing is an automatic process most of the time, but we can assume conscious command whenever we wish.

The brain control of *speaking* is as complicated as speech itself. Experts who have devoted a lifetime to research in brain functions are still in doubt about many details. For our practical purposes, a few facts that most of the scientists agree upon are sufficient.

To be able to speak, we need centers which receive outside messages. We hear the speech of others and relay the acoustical sensations to the brain by the pathways of hearing. The same happens to visual impressions, if we look at objects or at reading material. All of these incoming messages must be understood and interpreted. This takes place in the *sensory speech center,* or *auditory cortex,* located in the temple region of the brain, which was described first and named after the German psychiatrist Wernicke.

Then, with the help of other centers in the "thinking area" of the brain that store memories and promote associations, the message we intend to send out by the spoken word is prepared. Now, the actual act of speaking can begin. This requires the concerted effort of the many muscles that move the lips, tongue, palate, throat, vocal folds, and the machinery of breathing.

This complex mechanism is under the control of a *motor speech center* located in the frontal region of the brain surface. The French surgeon Paul Broca determined the localization of this center by a simple and ingenious method. In a number of patients who had shown loss of motor speech after a stroke, he looked, after the death of the patient, for the area of brain damage. He drew outlines of the brain and of the field of destruction on tracing paper. By putting a pile of such tracings on top of each other, he found that they all had in common a small area on the left side of the frontal brain and concluded that the center of speech movements must be located there.

To illustrate the whole process by a simple example, suppose somebody asks you how much two times two is. Your ears receive the sound of the words and telegraph the question as acoustic impressions to the brain where it is delivered to Wernicke's sensory speech center. With the help of other areas in the "thinking center," the question is understood, interpreted, the correct answer "four" prepared (by reviving schoolday memories), and finally relayed to Broca's motor speech center. Under its command, all your vocal organs begin at once to work as a team with the result that the answer is produced in the form of a spoken word.

The nerve fibers of the brain, on their way from the centers to the spinal cord and from there to the muscles, cross over to the other side. Thus, the left side of the brain serves the right side of the body and vice versa. In most people, speech is controlled on the left side of the brain. Damage to the motor regions of this side of the brain — for instance, by the internal bleeding of a stroke — has very tragic consequences. In addition to the loss of motion in the right arm or leg, the patient also will lose the ability to speak if Broca's center is involved.

---

*T*his has been a very sketchy outline of a complicated and highly controversial subject, but together with everything else we discussed in this chapter it will help to confirm the conviction expressed in the beginning — what a miracle the first word, the first sentence we speak really is. So many organs have to work in finest coordination to make speech possible that it is no wonder that speech is the privilege of man, the highest form of organized life on earth.

Speech originated as an instrument for simple communication. Early man must have been satisfied and proud to utter short sentences, expressing facts, reports, commands, desires, and emotions. The speech of mankind has grown through the eons. It has become a tool for innumerable uses. This variety of a fully developed instrument, the possibilities and requirements of its professional use, and the integration of voice and personality will be the subjects of the next chapter.

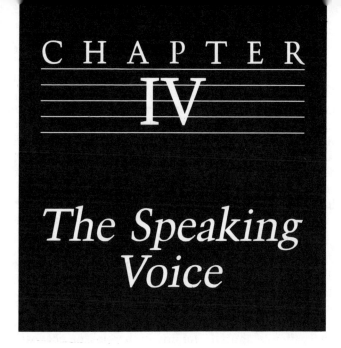

CHAPTER IV

The Speaking Voice

*O*ne of the advantages the student of the human voice enjoys is that he hardly ever gets bored if he listens to somebody else. Of course, he shares the common preference for the interesting, the entertaining, the witty fare for his ears. But even if the play is dull, the sermon overlong, the political speech full of platitudes, the radio program below his level, or the dinner conversation banal, he does not suffer too much. Unwilling to follow what is said, he concentrates on the "how." He analyzes voices.

To do so means to turn one of the greatest burdens of modern life into an enjoyable asset. For anyone who prefers to think his own thoughts, the flood of words that engulfs us everywhere, from loud-speakers, through windows and walls, is almost intolerable unless he develops some kind of escape mechanism. To analyze the "how" to escape from the "what" would have its own justification, but it is much more than an intellectual self-defense. Listening to voices can teach us a great deal about the speaker's background, social and professional standing, health, and personality.

To a certain degree, we all analyze voices without being aware of it. We speak of pleasant, sincere, affected, monotone, or irritating voices, but our judgment is based either on one outstanding voice symptom or on a general superficial impression.

The physician who specializes in voice disorders (known professionally as an otolaryngologist) and the speech and voice therapist
(known as the speech-language pathologist) have to learn to examine a
voice as the physician does the body, to consider each function
separately, take note of all deviations from the normal, and finally
synthesize all findings into one overall diagnosis.

The professional, seeing a voice patient for the first time, will let
the patient talk and read, watching all the time the "how" more than
the "what," and trying to ascertain a number of basic facts:

- The patient's general background, country of origin, regional
  characteristics, social level, educational and professional
  standing
- Basic features of his or her individual speech and voice
- Clues about personality
- The patient's aptitude for his or her job or occupation

All abnormalities of speech and voice are noted as the basis of our
diagnosis of the patient's troubles.

I hope to stimulate your interest in this kind of analytical hearing. No book can be substituted for the trained ear. By concentrated
listening to voices in conversation, on the radio, in movies and plays,
one can develop a high degree of judgment of people through analysis
of their voices if one knows where the clues are.

Much of the knowledge in this field has come from the study of
the disturbed voice. As in all branches of medicine, the abnormal is
often a good starting point for the understanding of normal function.

We like to think of ourselves as individuals, unique and different
from all others. Actually, we are, to a large extent, the products of our
surroundings. The country we belong to, the place where we live, our
social and professional background, our psychological type determine
countless details of our personality. Listening to speech teaches us a
great deal about these formative factors. It is often easy to determine
whether someone is speaking a native language or an adopted
language. Years ago an interesting radio program, run by an expert in
linguistics, enjoyed great popularity. By talking to guests for a few
minutes, he almost invariably was able to bring out their place of birth
within a radius of a few hundred miles, to tell them where they went
to college, and to trace their subsequent residential itinerary. The
farther removed we are from the residence of another person, the
more difficult it is for us to discover his or her personal speech and
voice habits under the layers of group characteristics. In Rome,
a tourist from Atlanta, Georgia will appear to Italian ears as an English speaking person. In London the same tourist will be immediately

identified as an American. In New York people will immediately recognize the Southern drawl; in Georgia her speech will stamp her as a city dweller. Only in Atlanta will she be on home ground with her voice. There, the individualities of her speech will stick out even for less well trained observers.

Social level, racial temperaments, professional surroundings, and many other influences leave their mark on speech and voice. What may be the expected pattern of one group would be abnormal in another. The speech and voice characteristics of a fisherman would be as incongruous in the mouth of a big-city lawyer as hunting clothes would be on Park Avenue.

---

*H*aving thus cleared away the group characteristics, we can turn to the analysis of the basic components of individual speech. A very good way of training one's ear to perceive the finer details of speech is to listen to the radio. There a great variety of disembodied voices is offered at all times with no visual crutches to help us in making our observations. Speech-language pathologists make frequent use of *recordings* of the voices of their patients. They can be played many times, permitting concentration on different features. The judgment of one therapist can be submitted to the critical review of others who have never seen the patient. Recordings can also be used to compare the voice or speech of the same individual at different times.

Analysis of a speaking voice includes appraisal of both articulation and voice. Outside of speech defects where, of course, the examination of all elements of articulation stands in the foreground, the importance of articulation is somewhat overrated. In judging speaking voices, voice deserve much more attention than it usually gets. In schools, training centers for teachers and ministers, and in drama departments, the qualities of the voice are too often neglected in favor of articulation, a heritage from the times when "elocutionists" taught an artificial declamatory style. Articulation carries only the factual contents of the spoken message, while voice conveys the whole gamut of emotions and the impact of personality.

With the neglect of voice culture in our education and training, it is no wonder that a clear, pleasant, and impressive voice has become a rarity and sticks out of the flood of deformed, distorted, and ill-fitting voices that surround us everywhere. It is characteristic that one good book on voice lists only the negative qualities one should watch for in speaking voices: breathy, harsh, hoarse, nasal. We hear them constantly.

In examining voices, one has to follow a certain routine. I still like to use an approach, introduced by Dr. P. Moses, which permits a systematic approach to the analysis of speaking voices. His scheme has the added advantage that it is easy to remember because the main terms all begin with an R. The five Rs are respiration, range, register, resonance, and rhythm.

We have met *respiration* frequently as the driving force of the voice. Every speaker has a characteristic way of breathing life into words. Whether we make conversation, address a crowd, recite Shakespearean periods, or tell an amusing story, our breathing can be adequate, fitted to the occasion, effortless, or pressed, exaggerated, and insufficient.

Respiration mirrors the emotional equilibrium at all times, as you probably have found out when you had to make your first speech. At home, in the quietude of your study, the sentences of your manuscript sounded fine when you tried them out. But on the stage, under the pressure of tension or stage fright, you were suddenly confronted with the problem of "catching" your breath for effective delivery. The inspiration-expiration rhythm can be upset one way or the other, being inadequate or using too much pressure, disrupting the message of the sentence.

Range comprises the deviations from the basic pitch that creates the melody of our speech. We discussed pitch in the last chapter. The range of our speaking voice normally constitutes the lower third of the whole compass we can employ in singing. In listening to individual voices, we have to watch both the basic pitch and the range. A voice may be pitched too high or too low; it may exhibit an unusually wide range or be limited to a level of flat monotony.

The change of our moods particularly influences basic pitch and range. In excitement or sudden fear, the pitch goes up and the range may widen, while depression lowers the pitch and narrows the range to a dull lifelessness.

I will have more to say in the next chapter about the *registers* of the singing voice. Suffice it to say here that the adult speaking voice is a blend of the deep, the chest register, and the high, the head register. I will discuss the change of voice in adolescence in the next chapter and the abnormalities of this process, which result in separation of the registers and the constant use of a wrong register, in Chapter XI.

Resonance, as we have seen before, is a basic function of voice production. Every change in the form and shape of the resonating cavities influences the quality and character of the voice sounds. The trained ear can detect many deviations from normal resonance and can even determine the exact place of tightness or weakness in the resonating cavities. An outstanding example of such a change of resonance is nasality of speech, which is caused by momentary or permanent relaxation (or paralysis) of the soft palate. The reasons for this occurrence are minifold, as we shall see.

Finally, the *rhythm* of speech is a rather complex phenomenon. Rhythm rules our life in many ways and finds its expression in speech too. The language we speak provides the basic rhythm, from the fast delivery of Spanish to the slow pace and hesitant groupings of words in English. Our station in life also puts its stamp on the speed, the duration of the individual sounds, and the groupings and stressing of words in our speech. The speech rhythm — and the rhythm of life — of a farmer and of a salesman are different. The small-town resident likewise differs from the big-city dweller, the minister from the lawyer, the slow-thinking from the quick-minded.

We shall meet all the basic features of speech again when we come to the discussion of voice and speech disturbances in the last part of the book. At this point, I just want to stress again the importance of getting away from generalized description of voices by terms which have no specific meaning and of learning to analyze each single factor that goes into the making of a voice.

---

*B*ecause voice is one of the functions most characteristic of an individual, this question leads us logically to the connection between voice and personality.

Dr. P. Moses, whom I mentioned earlier, believed that it is possible, by "creative hearing," to find out a great deal about an individual's personality and personality problems. By watching closely every detail of the speaking voice, a compositive picture emerges of personality traits, moods, attitudes and many other facets of the personality. As in all studies of human psychology, great experience is required to pick the really important data out of a mass of detail and to assign the correct significance to each symptom. One difficulty in identifying the meaning of each observable symptom lies in the fact that it is frequently what the psychologists call ambivalent, it can be interpreted in a positive or a negative way.

A man who speaks in a slow rhythm may be sure of himself, thinking carefully before he ventures an opinion, and weighing his words before he lets them out, or he may be slow of speech because he is slow of thinking, dull-witted, or shy and hesitant. Or he may affect this mode of speaking out of an exaggerated opinion of his own importance, speaking constantly in pronunciamentos to which everybody should pay close attention. In short, he may be a born leader, a stupid man, or a pompous ass. Rapid speech, on the other hand, may be the expression of a mind overflowing with ideas or just the mirror of a shallow personality that releases a stream of superficial small talk without inhibition or criticism.

In the field of voice disturbances, knowledge of the voice-personality relationship can be a great help to better understanding of the causes of such conditions. Take, for instance, a person with a rather deep speaking voice. This will be his or her natural pitch if he or she belongs to the class of bassos. It may be the expression of great authority. The preacher, the judge, the doctor, the king on the stage, anyone who represents authority, tends to speak with the true pathos of deep sonorous voices. Such people will have no voice troubles since they use their voices at a genuine pitch, fitting the personality and the occasion.

But if I see a patient with voice trouble such as hoarseness after short periods of speaking and note that his or her voice is produced on an abnormally deep level, I have to consider a number of possible causes: chronic laryngitis and other organic causes, lack of tension or weakness of the folds, glandular imbalances. But I will also keep in mind the possibility that the patient has lowered his or her voice, consciously or subconsciously, to create the impression of authority he actually does not possess. Young ministers, teachers, and district attorneys are frequently the victims of using this lower register as a means of concealing their inner immaturity or conveying an impression of authority.

A loud voice may be the expression of energy and confidence as well as the product of a primitive mind without self-criticism. The absence or exaggeration of nasality is another indicator of moods and emotions. A group of doctors at the New York Hospital published the results of an extremely interesting study of the influence of emotions on the mucous membranes of the nose and the deeper respiratory tract.[*] By observing their patients closely for months, they showed that any change in the patient's mood, any increase or decrease of tensions, fears, or apprehensions is paralleled by the obstruction or widening of nasal passages, bronchi, and bronchioles. It stands to reason that such changes influence voice resonance and vary the degree of nasality.

I could go on like this — and the temptation is great — for a long time without exhausting all possibilities. I would have to speak of melody of speech, exactness, accents and stresses, and many other

---

[*] Holmes, T. H., Goodell, H., Wolf, S., and Wolff, Y. H. 1950. *The nose.* Springfield, Illinois: Charles C Thomas.

features of the speaking voice. The limited selection I have presented should be sufficient to impress three facts on you:

- That there exists an intimate connection between voice and personality, emotional balance, moods, and passing and lasting emotions.
- That a correct interpretation can be reached only with great care, by consideration not of one single outstanding symptom but only by a synthetic evaluation of all available details. This requires great experience and understanding. Psychological analysis of the personality by any approach is not the intellectual parlor game by which it is so frequently abused these days.
- That — with these limitations in mind — listening to voices can teach us a great deal.

Vocal analysis is a new and very promising field. Many questions still need to be answered, much research needs to be done on a large scale, many doubts need to be cleared away; but in the end, we may be able to prove that vocal analysis is a valuable tool for understanding the human mind.

---

*N*ow let us turn to a subject of immediate practical application, the specific requirements for the different uses of speech and voice. Too little attention has been paid to this subject. Every year, thousands of young people embark on careers that are founded on the use of the voice without giving a thought — or even being advised to get an opinion — on their aptitude for such work. It cannot be emphasized too much that everybody at this crossroad of life should get a complete checkup by a competent examiner. The vocal organs should be investigated for all kinds of possible organic abnormalities, such as obstructions of the nose, sinus troubles, adenoids, tonsillitis, allergies, and asthma. The larynx should be inspected and the shape, appearance, motility, and closure of the vocal folds should be determined. Finally, and most important of all, speech and voice should be tested by an expert who has been trained in this field and knows something about the working conditions of the voice in jobs and professions. In this respect, very little work has been done. Aptitude tests almost invariably omit consideration of the voice.

Take the case of salespeople, for instance. The big department stores test their permanent employees carefully, train them in preparatory courses, but pay no attention to the correct and efficient use of the voice. If you go through the busy sections of a large store, you can hear all kinds of bad voices. Salespeople, who often talk almost incessantly in noisy surroundings for eight hours a day, five days a week, easily develop voice troubles from constant abuse, pressure, and strain. If you start your career in this field with poor speech and voice habits, you are a likely candidate for permanent disturbances.

The higher the qualities of goods to be sold, the greater the need for the persuasiveness of a pleasant voice. You need more than great stamina that can produce quantities of speech without getting tired or hurt. It is the quality of a good sales voice — a voice which expresses your interest in your work — that counts. What makes us so often buy things we did not intend to? It is, as most employers believe (aside from the desirability of the object), the sales talk, the "what," or is it the influence of the voice, the "how"? One thing is certain, the over-worked, overstrained voices we hear so often in stores and office make us uncomfortable and create the wish to get out of earshot as fast as possible.

Switchboard operators, with their long hours of constant talk, work under the handicap of quantity too. In this type of work, clear-ness of articulation, of course, counts, but good voice is essential for success. The big telephone companies know that very well. They are almost the only employers who put candidates for jobs through sys-tematic training of speech and voice. In addition, they have created large laboratories where extensive research is done on acoustic and phonetic problems.

Next to sales personnel and telephone operators, *teachers* of all kinds carry the heaviest load of speaking. Teaching puts a great strain on the voice, by the sheer quantity of speech alone. Teachers have to represent authority in front of a class that is often resistant, noisy, and even belligerent. If they are born educators with natural authority and a sound voice, their job is not too difficult. But only a minority can fulfill all these requirements. The result is frequently the use of a voice that is out of focus in pitch, function, and economy. Voice troubles are a typical occupational hazard of the teacher. Still, aside from watching faults of articulation, very little is done in the training of teachers to study and improve their voices. This is more regrettable because teachers set standards by their own examples. Their pupils pick up faulty speech and voice habits from them while their own voices are still in the formative stage. In addition, the resistance we all feel if exposed to unpleasant and irritating voices endangers the relationship between teacher and pupil. To watch and correct faults of articulation of teachers in training is not enough. Nobody should be permitted to choose the teaching profession without an examination and, if necessary, correction of his voice.

The higher the standards of professional speech are — both in content and delivery — in any type of work, the less important the tolerance for great quantities of speech becomes and the more decisive the quality of speech becomes. In professions such as the minister's, the lawyer's, the actor's, the lecturer's, psychological factors create special voice hazards. The tension, the responsibilities, the risks, and the personnel problems combine to throw the speaker off balance emotionally. The importance of voice for success in these careers exposes professional users of voice to the dangers of vocal hypochondria; and the neurotic conflicts so frequently seen in these professions have a preference for fixation on the voice.

As with the teachers, guidance in the use of the voice should form a main subject in the training of *ministers*. What they actually get is very little or nothing. Any speech-language pathologist who has worked with divinity students knows that their first sermons are very often quite an ordeal. Some ministers — even widely known stars of the pulpit — fight with their voices through their whole lives. Nobody analyzed their vocal equipment when they began to study. They have to speak in churches and temples with obstinate acoustics. The burden of representing moral authority in the upheavals and contradictions of modern society is rather heavy.

The voice troubles of ministers are less often the result of a cold or laryngitis than they are the expression of poor training, faulty use, and constant strain of the vocal organs. Expert guidance and advice during the years of training would go far to eradicate this scourge of the clerical profession.

While the minister uses voice to guide people, the task of *actors* is to imitate and recreate life in all its forms. This requires a tremendous flexibility and adaptability of the voice, which only a few achieve. In addition, they have to master the technique of "projection," the ability to bridge the distance — sometimes very great — between stage and the audience without changing or distorting the type of speech the play requires. A perfect speaking voice will be equally natural, audible, and pleasant to your ears whether you sit in the first row of the orchestra or high up in the balcony. Clarity of diction helps a great deal, but the good use of the voice, equally well adapted to the character of the part as to the acoustic dimensions of the theater, decides the success.

In our age of mass communications nobody can escape the influence of television and radio. The overexcited, overstrained voices that reach us constantly set new patterns and fashions of speech and voice, particularly with the younger generation. The messages of the media are conveyed through microphone and loudspeaker. One could write a whole book about the microphone, its impact on modern society, its possibilities and limitations, and its effect on human voices. The microphone has narrower limits in range and intensity than the human voice. If you speak through a microphone — as actor, politician, lecturer, preacher — you should be thoroughly familiar with the technique it requires. You must be able to express the whole variety of emotions while respecting the limits of loudness where distortion or lack of response begin. Most radio speaking is done with directional microphones which are sensitive to any change of the position of the speaker. A turn of the head or a step to the side changes the effect of the voice for the listener.

The microphone has radically changed the impact of the human voice on our political life. It has become both a blessing and curse. It has made possible the "fireside chat" where a voice can talk to millions in conversational tones. And it has served as a tool in the creation of mass hysteria by the voice of one man alone. Modern dictatorships have rediscovered the truth of a remark Gibbon made 175 years ago, that "the mechanical operation of sounds, by quickening of the blood and spirits, will act on the human machine more forcibly than the eloquence of reason and honor."

Those of us who put the microphone to more peaceful pursuits easily overlook the effect of this mechanization of sound on the quality of the human voice. If we speak through a microphone, the listener does not hear our voice but hears a filtrate of our voice sounds through the medium of a complicated machinery. Apart from the distortion which poor equipment produces, we are at the mercy of the sound engineer. This modern Pygmalion can create voices, out of almost nothing, by the witchcraft of her panel. She can blow up conversational speech to the dimensions of the arena. She can speed up, slow down, or mechanically emphasize a particular frequency, thereby changing the character of a voice completely. We have seen how important the overtones, which range through the whole compass of audible sounds, are to the quality and expressivity of the voice sounds we produce.

Finally, the microphone has become a crutch that threatens to destroy the art of free speaking. Most speakers have become so dependent on the assistance of the microphone that they are afraid to address a hundred listeners without it. Movie and television actors have lost the ability to project their voices and go through agonies when they want to appear in a play.

It is time that we learn again to use the natural force and power of our voices as did our fathers who thought nothing of speaking for an hour to an audience of a thousand and more without microphones. If we can do that only by reducing the daily flow of speech which engulfs us now to rarer and more important occasions, we can only benefit from such rationing of words.

Of course, power and force can be overdone. The auctioneer, and the barker at the country fair have to put a prolonged strain on their voices. Only few vocal folds can sustain it with impunity. In this category the *voice of command* ranks high as particularly dangerous. The soldier who leads men has to use loud voice in short powerful bursts. His commands have to be sharp in articulation and clearly audible on the drill ground as well as in the field. They must carry the ring of absolute authority which men follow without questioning even under danger of life. The easiest but rather dangerous way of producing the penetrating command voice is to use the so-called *glottal stroke,* the forceful compression of the vocal folds which permits the explosive release of pent-up air. This leads to thickening of the folds or to the formation of nodes which, in turn, necessitate even greater force for loud commands. The "fog-horn" voices of the top sergeant, and of the oldtime sailing ship captain are sad examples of the ruining of voices by long abuse.

Military training schools should include instruction in the proper use of the voice in their curriculum. Instead of insisting on harsh barking, the proper technique of starting with a soft attack and of stepping up sound in rapidly increasing volume — the way a good driver operates the gas pedal — should be taught.

There are many more different types of professional work requiring voice and speech, each with its own characteristic tasks and voice problems. Altogether, it should be clear — even from this short survey — that no simple prescription can be given for a good speaking voice. The most important requirement for everybody who uses speech in his or her work is to retain and develop his or her normal voice. Very few of us manage to escape the distorting influences of modern life. Voices of normal pitch, melody, and flexibility are as rare as normal feet in our shoe-ridden civilization.

The only way out of this deplorable situation is *preventive voice care* on the largest scale. Systematic training of teachers, examination and care of adolescent voices, and advice before and during job and professional training would go a long way to prevent the damage to voices we experience now everywhere.

So far, we have bypassed the finest use to which the human voice can be applied, artistic singing. It deserves a chapter of its own.

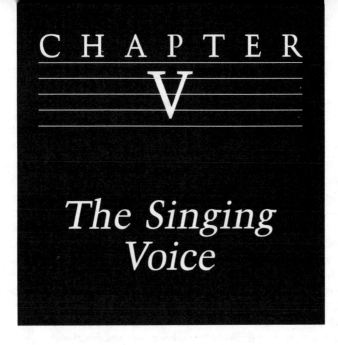

CHAPTER V

The Singing Voice

A few can touch the magic string,
And noisy Fame is proud to win them: —
Alas for those that never sing,
But die with all their music in them!

O f the many thoughtful lines that Oliver Wendell Holmes, doctor and writer of "Autocrat" fame, has penned about the human voice, none have defined so simply the variability of the use of the singing voice from the release of the inner music in song by most of us to the glories of artistic singing by a chosen few.

We begin to sing almost as soon as we learn to speak. In an artless childish treble we imitate the songs of our mothers. They have to be simple to fit our narrow range. The best we can do at our second year is to produce a compass of six half-tones. Slowly the range widens.

According to Dr. E. Froeschels who measured the range of hundreds of school children, the normal range at six years reaches from b to a^1, at eight from a to c^2, at ten from g to d^2, at twelve from e to d^2 (almost two octaves). The big change comes with puberty. Up to then, the voices of boys and girls follow the same line. *Mutation,* as the *change of voice* is called, is the crossroads where male and female voices separate. During puberty, the fast-maturing sex glands release hormones into the bloodstream and stimulate the development of the secondary sex characteristics that distinguish the adult body from the child's. The change of voice is but one of the manifestations of this stormy period. In temperate zones it takes place in girls between twelve and fourteen years and in boys between thirteen and fifteen. In warmer climates it begins one to two years earlier, in the cold zones up to two years later.

The slow growth of the larynx in childhood is suddenly accelerated in puberty. The cartilages extend, mostly in the anterior-posterior direction. The Adam's apple assumes its prominence, the neck lengthens, and the larynx moves to the middle of the neck. The vocal folds grow by about two-fifths of an inch in the male and by one-eighth of an inch in the female. At the end of mutation the lower limit of the male voice has descended by an average of an octave while the upper limit has dropped by a sixth. In girls, both limits descend only one to two tones.

In the majority of boys the whole process develops very gradually with no appreciable break of the voice. Only a small percentage go through the period of cracking or breaking voice. In these cases, the change might come almost overnight and throw the coordination of the vocal muscles completely out of gear. For instance, a former president of Radio Corporation of America used to sing in a synagogue choir as a boy of fifteen with a fine soprano voice. On the day before the High Holidays, when he expected to earn one hundred dollars for his singing, his voice suddenly broke, depriving him of much-needed income. This sudden end to a vocal career started him on a career in business, for which he later became famous.

No certain prognosis can be made from a boy's voice about the quality and type of voice that he will develop. A child's soprano often becomes a baritone or basso, while altos frequently develop into tenors. Caruso sang alto in a church choir. Chaliapin was a soprano before mutation.

While the speaking voice settles in an average of three to six months, with one year being the extreme limit for normal development, the singing voice needs much more time for full development. This is of practical importance for the answer to a question we have to discuss very often with our patients: At what age can serious vocal studies be safely begun?

In this connection, a discussion has raged for hundreds of years whether or not singing should be permitted at all during the change of voice. Manuel Garcia fought for complete voice rest against Dr. Morel MacKenzie, who believed that easy exercises would be helpful in the transition of the voice. But all experts agree that choir singing — the prevalent form of singing at that age — with its lack of individual control is very harmful. Schubert and Hayden lost their voices that way. Serious vocal studies should not be begun by boys before the age of eighteen to nineteen, by girls before seventeen.

The adult voice has a range of at least two octaves, but many trained voices extend over three octaves and more. We have to distinguish between physiological and musical range. While the first includes all notes that can be produced by a person, the latter is limited to the range of artistically satisfactory sounds.

By old tradition, male voices are classified as bassos, baritones, and tenors; female voices as contraltos (and altos), mezzo-sopranos, and sopranos (Figure V-1). The basic speaking pitch — marked by small horizontal lines — corresponds closely to the range of the singing voice. As we shall see later, any marked discrepancy between voice type and speaking pitch of great significance in voice disturbances.

The absolute range is greater in deep voices. Bassos have the widest range, tenors the smallest, with baritones standing in the middle. The same relations, but to a lesser degree, are found in female voices. Of course, one should always keep in mind that these figures are average, and that all such classifications are artificial. Really deep bassos — the *basso absoluto* of the Italians — and high tenors, and true contraltos are very rare. The majority of voices are found in the middle ranges.

To determine the true character of a voice is one of the oldest and most difficult problems of the singing teacher. It is not made any easier by the powerful lure of the extremes. Since a heavy premium in glory and money is placed on very high or very low voices, the temptation to extend the natural range in these directions is great. Many baritones have ruined their voices by masquerading as tenors, many a mezzo-soprano invaded the sopranos' territory to discover, too late, that one cannot leap over natural barriers with impunity. Some singers manage to just go by, others pay the price later. Chaliapin was actually not a basso but a deep baritone and ran into considerable voice difficulties in his maturer years. Some of the most famous contraltos of our time are actually mezzo-sopranos, and the early deterioration of their voices is a sad commentary on overextension of range. But the audiences roar if a singer hits the deep A or a high f^2, and nobody likes to think of the dangers of the future.

Aside from typing voices according to their ranges, we can classify them as to their character. The *dramatic* and the *lyric* voices represent different types, in both voice and personality of the singer. Siegried and Don Octavio, Eleonore and Countess Almaviva not only pose very different vocal problems but ask for completely different personalities as well. The *buffi* have to be good comic actors and need

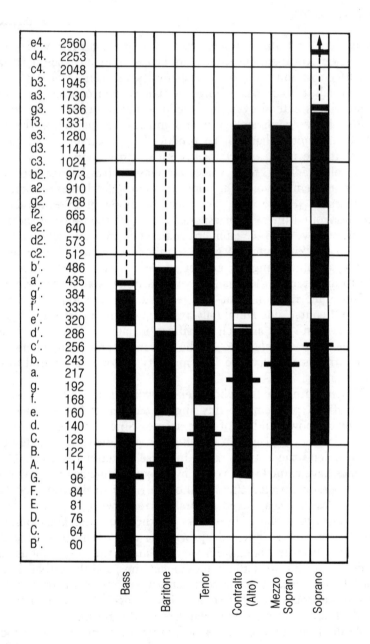

Figure V-1. *The ranges of the human voice. The gaps in the black bars indicate the approximate position of the transitions between registers. The dotted areas above the bass, baritone, and tenor bars are the falsetto ranges. The dotted area above the soprano voice marks the whistle register. The horizontal lines that extend out from the bars indicate the average pitch of the speaking voice. [From Dr. M. Nadolesczny]*

flexible voices that permit a maximum of characterization. The true coloraturas are in a class by themselves. We shall discuss them when we come to the significance of registers.

Just in passing, I should like to mention another type of voice that belongs to history: the *castrati*. The seventeenth and eighteenth centuries were the time of their greatest triumphs. Someone has figured that during that era in Italy four thousand boys were castrated every year to produce singers for the growing demands of church choirs and opera houses. Singing with the larynx of a child and the chest power of an adult, trained to a technical brilliance that will never again be duplicated, they were the greatest stars of their time. They made the Sistine Chapel Choir in Rome world famous; singers like Caffarelli, Farinelli, Senesino, and Bernacchi commanded fees that would make our tenors blanch with envy. The *Orpheus* (Monteverdi and Gluck) and *Idomeneo* (Mozart) were written for castrati. Handel offered fabulous salaries to famous castrati for parts in his operas. With their passing from the musical scene, the age of greatest singing came to a close to be followed by a new conception that valued dramatic truth in opera higher than smoothness of technique.

To succeed in opera today is the ambition of many singers. Too often, the satisfaction of concert work is overlooked. In many European countries, the artist who excels in the art of the lied, the oratorio, is valued as highly as the operatic star (although the income is usually smaller). Music in America is relatively young. With the tremendous expansion of concert life in the last twenty years, we have begun to rely less on big opera stars and more on artists who master the different style of the concert hall. This is a very healthy symptom of our musical growth and one that will give new opportunities to many young artists. A very strange by-product of modern mass communications is the *microphone voice* that becomes famous overnight and fades away after a short burst of a very profitable popularity. The majority of these so-called "voices," which sell millions of records, are artificial creations of the amplifier that would sound tinny and shaky if the stars ever tried to sing without clutching a microphone.

Thousands of singers who do not make the grade in opera and concert work as *soloists* in *church choirs*. This can be a very satisfactory occupation, both artistically and — on a modest level — economically. It is steady work, a rarity in the arts. It requires a great amount of musicality and versatility, and an easy facility in sight-reading.

Can the *type of voice* be *determined by physical examination?* Teachers and singers have asked this question very often and, as usual, the experts disagree. Certain rules have been established, but exceptions can be quoted to each of them. The singer is the instrument and the instrumentalist at the same time, and it stands to reason that body structure should reflect the character of the voice as do instruments, for instance, the violin and the cello.

To begin with the vocal folds, definite characteristics exist. Most singers with low voices have long and relatively thin folds, while those with high voices have short and broad folds. The coloraturas sometimes have an incredibly small larynx with very short vocal folds.

The whitest folds are found in tenors and high sopranos, while those of deep voices usually have a more pinkish tinge. Dr. D. Weiss, who examined a large number of successful singers, believes that a definite body type can be associated with the high and low voices. According to him, singers with high voices have round faces with short noses, a convex profile with small delicate details, short necks, round or quadratic chests, and high palates with delicate soft palates; while the deep voices are characterized by long faces with long noses, straight-line profiles with massive details, long and narrow necks, long and flat chests, and broad palates with massive soft palates. A flat palate or a sharp angle between the floor of the mouth and the neck was rarely found in a singer with a good voice. As long as we have not established these characteristics as certain, it would be dangerous to design voices by physical characteristics alone. Still, it is astonishing how many singers fit into this schema if one analyzes their body structure.

Fundamentally, singing is the same regardless of the purpose or grade. Whether we "sing" with our vocal folds in the speaking voice, or produce our best "bathroom tenor," our vocal organs follow the same basic laws of acoustics as the larynx of a Caruso. There is no need to repeat here the explanations of laryngeal function we gave in Chapter II. I want to limit our discussion to a few facts that pertain to *artistic singing*.

With *respiration* being the driving power of the larynx, good breathing is the basis of perfect singing. Artistic singing requires the ability to sing long musical phrases with all of the accents and changes in intensity and pitch that the composer provided. No simple formula can be given that would fit all voices. Graphic records of the chest and abdominal breathing of famous singers of the same voice category show great differences in the breathing mechanism. It is the task of the teacher to find out for each individual student by what teamwork of chest and abdomen the goal of every good singer can best be reached: to sing with the greatest economy of air. The less air used for a certain sound — whether piano or forte — the better the result will be.

This minimum consumption of air is possible only if all air is transformed into sound waves. Any attempt to obtain uncertain notes by enforced breathing — one of the most common faults of technique — will only lead to *waste of air,* the audible escape of unutilized air through the folds that is equally as detrimental to esthetic result as to the health of the voice. A good singer can sing a note without producing a flicker in the flame of a candle in front of the mouth.

Excessive wavering of the voice — up to twelve times per second — is called *tremolo,* a greatly feared symptom of poor or deteriorating voices. It happens frequently in "throaty" voices and may be due to overtenseness of the muscles, which creates a vibrating trembling in the throat, the tongue, and sometimes even the jaw.

One factor that influences singing voices gravely is not so well known, the *standard pitch* used in tuning the instruments of the orchestra. If we read a score by Bach or Mozart, we usually assume that the notes they wrote are the same we hear today when their works are performed. Actually, pitch has constantly risen in the last three hundred years. The old organ builders in the seventeenth century were the first to raise the standard pitch (Diapason) of the a^1 in order to save material by shorter pipes. From their pitch of 375-400, the a^1 rose at the time of Mozart and Handel to 420. In the nineteenth century the pitch became still higher, until in 1859 a French commission fixed the "diapason normal" at 435 double vibrations per second (now known as "Hertz"). While all of Europe accepted this as standard pitch, the English continued to force the pitch until it had reached the peak of 458. The famous German violinist Joseph Joachim complained that he had to start tuning up his violin eight weeks before a concert in London to prevent injury to the instrument by a sudden change.

Finally, an international agreement fixed the standard pitch at 435. This figure is still used in most textbooks although in the meantime a new change has taken place. Unfortunately, in the last twenty-five years orchestras, especially in America, have again raised the pitch because it gives the woodwinds and, to a lesser degree, the other instruments a greater degree of brilliance. We now hold at 440, which was accepted in 1939 by an international conference in London. The U.S. Bureau of Standards in Washington, D.C., broadcasts daily a radio signal of 440 Hertz as a standard a^1.

Smooth teamwork of the chest and abdominal breathing characterize all good voices. Marked reliance on one type of breathing is almost always the sign of a poor technique that leads sooner or later to voice disturbances. The enforced chest breathing with lifting of the shoulders at the height of inspiration is particularly dangerous. It is a signal for the need of speedy correction before irreparable damage is done to the voice.

A great confusion surrounds the term *breathing support.* The support, or as the Italians call it, the *appoggio,* is a special technique of slowing down the rate of expiration. Unfortunately, as it so often happens in discussions of singing, body sensations have been confused with the mechanics of function. Teachers have spoken of inspirational tension, or have claimed the forehead or the nose as the seat of the support for the voice.

We still cannot completely explain support in scientific terms. This much is certain: in true support the expiration is artificially slowed down by clinging as long as possible, after expiration has begun, to the position at the end of inspiration. Either the chest or the abdominal wall is kept at an extended position while the counterpart begins to contract. The abdominal support — leaving the abdominal wall and the flanks extended during the first phase of inspiration — is generally considered the preferred method, and has been observed in top-ranked Italian singers. The "inspirational tension" that has been described by teachers and singers is a body sensation which should not be confused with the demonstrable slowing down of expiration that actually takes place. Expiration — whether slow or fast — is necessary for any kind of singing.

The use of subjective body sensations has a legitimate place in teaching. The student is often helped more by explanations in terms of such sensations than by physiological discourse, but the teacher who has to know the functional facts should always keep in mind that a valid analysis of the mechanics of singing can be given only in terms of graphs, curves, or by other means of scientific registration and observation.

Next to support no other detail of singing technique has suffered so much from misinterpretation as the term *register.* For generations, singers, teachers, and doctors have formulated so many different explanations and classifications of registers that it is difficult to find a way through the maze of theories. Modern experimental research has brought some clarification, but Manuel Garcia, who did not have our laboratory equipment, still presented one of the best definitions. In his *Traité Complet de L'Art du Chant* written in 1841, he said: "By the word register we mean a series of succeeding sounds of equal quality on a scale from high to low, produced by the application of the same mechanical principle, the nature of which differs basically from another series of succeeding sounds of equal quality produced by another mechanical principle. Consequently, all the sounds which belong to the same register are of the same nature, regardless of changes in pitch or force which they are submitted."

If a person with an untrained voice sings a downward scale from a high note, two breaks will be heard, marking the limits of three different registers: the head, the middle, and the chest register. The same occurs, of course, on an upward scale. On a descending scale, the breaks occur at deeper points than on an ascending one. For the experienced ear, each group of sounds has a different quality.

It is the purpose of any training of voice to make these transitional breaks disappear and to blend the whole range into one smooth unit. In a good voice it requires great practice to hear the transitions from one register to another. In the chart of Figure V-1 you find the average points of transition marked by small white spaces in the black columns.

High-speed cinematography has thrown some light on the registers. In the chest register, the whole mass of the folds vibrates rhythmically, while in the head register only the inner margins of the highly tensed folds participate in the vibrations. At the same time, the posterior parts of the folds remain firmly closed — the damping effect that prevents vibration so that only the anterior halves or thirds are left free to vibrate in the inner margins.

Ideal singing is done in a mixture of register characteristics — a *voix mixte.* Each tone of the compass receives a little of the color of the opposing registers in a mixture that varies from equal parts in the middle of the range to heavier coloring at the extreme ends. The only case where a pure register is used in perfect singing is the coloratura, who sings in a clear head register.

The chest voice uses more air than the head voice. The complete vibration of the whole mass of the folds requires a higher pressure of air to produce sounds of equal intensity as in the head register. In the chest voice, the resonance can be felt in the breastbone. The vibrations in the chest have given the name to this register.

Male voices have on top of the head register the *falsetto* which, even to the untrained ear, has a distinctive quality of its own. The Italian masters of the early Bel Canto thought of it as an unnatural and, therefore, false voice — thence the name. Falsetto is sung with only the foremost parts of the folds left free to vibrate at the margins, the rest being damped (see Figure II-3C). It has less brilliance than the sounds of the head register. It can be used occasionally, but its continuous employment gives the voice an effeminate character.

Female voices have no real counterpart to the male falsetto, but the sopranos have a so-called *whistle register* on top of the head register (see Figure V-1). It has a shrill quality when used forte and sounds like a flute when piano. In artistic singing, it is used only in high, fast staccato notes as in the f^3 of the "Queen-of-the-Night" aria in the *Magic Flute.* (By some coincidence, Mozart's father Leopold was the first to describe this register.) Like the falsetto, the whistle register is produced by marginal vibration in the anterior third of the folds which leave a tiny elliptic chink open.

In 1836, a French tenor, Gilbert Duprez, appeared in Paris with a new singing method he learned in Italy. In 1840, two doctors, Diday and Pérequin described this technique calling it *voix sombrée, voix fermée,* or *voix couverte.* The last name stuck and because the *covered voice* in English. The controversy about the nature, the artistic value, and the advisability of covered singing has been raging ever since. Many details are still obscure. Hundreds of papers have been written about it, but only lately — thanks to modern methods of sound analysis — have we begun to understand a little better the nature of covering.

The experienced ear can detect the degree of covering by the peculiar color it gives to the voice. It sounds somewhat darker and, at the same time, more penetrating. It is, therefore, particularly suited to singing with great dramatic expression. Wagnerian singers usually employ extensive covering of the voice. Under the influence of Wagner, Richard Strauss, and the modern composers, covering has become, to a certain extent, the trademark of a German singer. The French do not like it much, and the Italians hate it. They prefer the *voce bianca,* the open voice. Play records of some great Wagnerian singer and of a first-class Italian singer in succession, and you will hear the difference in the vocal approach.

Covering has to be used with great care because, in its extreme form, it is hard on voices. Measurements of air volume have shown that the same note sung by the same singer uses up to double the amount of air in covered voice that it uses in open singing. The reason for this lies in the greater tension of the outer laryngeal muscles as well as of the inner ones both of which tense the folds.

The larynx is pulled downward in covering, while in open singing, it rises and falls with the pitch (although exceptions from this rule have been observed). Generally speaking, excessive movements of the larynx are typical of untrained or poor voices. In a mature singer, they are a danger symptom, at least, if the larynx moves in extreme, abrupt movements with the rise and fall of the pitch. The better trained the voice, the smaller the changes in position of the larynx in singing from low to high or vice versa.

In the last chapter I mentioned the *coup de glotte* or *glottal stroke.* The term is used to describe the hard attack of a note by sudden forceful compression of the folds with an explosive release of air. It is one of the most pernicious habits a singer can acquire, leading to formation of nodes, thickening of the folds, and hemorrhages into the folds.

The singer has to learn to attack even the most powerful fortissimo with a soft beginning. In high-speed cinematography the difference can be clearly seen. In soft attack, the folds begin to vibrate before they come in contact with each other. In the glottal stroke, the folds are squeezed together with frightening force until they are suddenly blown apart by the mounting air pressure. Even strong vocal folds cannot stand this treatment for any length of time without suffering serious and often irreparable damage.

There is one exception to the general condemnation of the glottal stroke. In *staccato* singing, a form of glottal stroke is used to produce the sharp interruptions of the sound that characterize it. But in good staccato the glottal stroke which starts each note is well controlled and done with a minimum of pressure to avoid damage to the folds.

A well-trained voice always exhibits a certain amount of *vibrato* that gives the sounds more life and expression. By vibrato, we mean small rhythmical changes, both in pitch and volume. These oscillations of no more than half a tone and two to three decibels are more noticeable in forte tones than in piano. They take place at the rate of about six to seven per second.

The sufferers of this development are the singers. Instruments can be tuned or built to conform to a higher pitch, but the human vocal folds remain the same. Mozart and Beethoven are played and have to be sung almost a half a tone higher than the composers heard it. The b^2 flat that Leonore has to throw with full force at the threatening Pizarro, the c^3 that rings through the end of Constance's big aria, and many similar hurdles of the operatic race course are now even more neck-breaking than they used to be for the singers of a more considerate time.

With the exception of the contraltos, all singers would be in favor of returning to the classical pitch. Audiences would benefit too, since they would be exposed to less of the shrieking we hear now so often. There is hardly a chance to reverse a trend that has become universally accepted. But, at least, singers should unite in putting a stop to any further attenpts to raise the standard pitch. No brilliance of the orchestra can compensate for the ruin of voices that follows each new upward change of pitch.

Now that you have a good grounding in the basics of speaking and singing, we can move on to the abnormalities that can affect the voice and the treatment of these conditions.

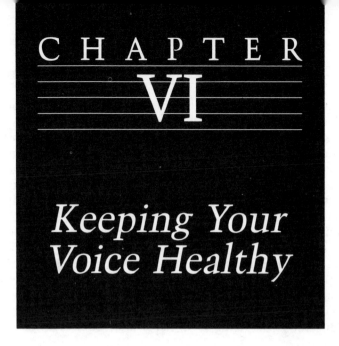

CHAPTER VI

Keeping Your Voice Healthy

*T*he Greeks had a word for it, and we still use it today. *Hygiene,* the science which deals with the preservation of health, has become a powerful force in the age-old struggle of mankind for a longer and happier life.

In the public domain, the rules of hygiene, as enforced by ordinances and regulations, health departments, and the medical profession, govern countless aspects of our daily lives and, with few exceptions, we cooperate. Yet, when it comes to personal hygiene, quite a different situation prevails. Years of study of patients and people in general have convinced me that personal hygiene consists, to a large extent, of advice freely given and rarely followed. And, as a rule, those who dispense the advice are not much better in living according to their own teachings.

To no group should the preservation of physical health be more important than to the men and women who make professional use of their speaking and singing voices. They are more vulnerable to any impairment of the vocal organs in particular; and due to the nature of their work which brings them into constant contact with large numbers of people, they are more susceptible to infections in general than the rest of us. Furthermore, the risk of temporary or permanently debilitating effects of sickness becomes greater as specialization in the use of the voice increases.

Sales people, lawyers, doctors, and the teachers, even ministers, will find it relatively easy to use their voices adequately in spite of a bad cold. The position of those in the acting profession is more precarious. But with voice training of sufficiently high caliber they may be able to go through their performances even though handicapped by a respiratory infection.

Among those who make professional use of their voices, the singer, above all, must practice intelligent hygiene. Without good general health and intactness of all vocal organs, execution of his or her art is impossible. This knowledge, unfortunately, often leads to a preoccupation with the health of the voice, which is dangerous in itself. Finding the proper middle course between sensible precautions and dangerous pampering is difficult and requires a lot of common sense.

In this chapter we are dealing with the problems of preserving health and preventing disease, with special emphasis on perfect functioning of the vocal organs. Since the speaking and singing voice can be put to a great variety of uses, no one simple set of rules can be laid down regarding intelligent hygiene. While ordinary precaution may be sufficient in many instances, a regime affecting all phases of daily life may be necessary in others.

I will refer to singers rather frequently, inasmuch as this profession requires the highest degree of specialization in the use of the voice. Singers stand to gain the most by following a strict program of daily hygiene. If you belong to one of the less sensitive groups, I trust that you will take my advice with a grain of salt.

To a large extent, preservation of health means the prevention of disease. One of the reasons for the vulnerability of the vocal organs lies in the fact that, by an unhappy coincidence, they form one of the frontiers on which the daily battle against disease is fought. In a way, the whole respiratory tract — nose, mouth, larynx, trachea, bronchi — belongs to the surface of the body. It forms an extension of the surface into the depths of the body, like the pockets of a suit. While our skin is reasonably tough and not easily penetrated by invading germs and viruses, the mucous membranes which line all vocal organs are delicate and vulnerable.

On the subject of vocal hygiene modern textbooks teach hardly any more than do the books that were written in the days of antiquity. Quintilian, the Roman author of *De Institutione Oratorica*, the first work on the art of public speaking, advised his readers to lead a simple life, to eat sensibly, and to get plenty of rest and sleep, a recommendation that need hardly be improved upon. Even lozenges, gargles, medicated fluids, licorice, and turpentine, so popular with singers and speakers in this age of patent medicines, were already being used.

During the Middle Ages, denial of bodily needs and comforts was regarded as a virtue, and in the field of vocal hygiene those days were dark ones too. Since the beginning of the Renaissance, however, with the singer and speaker gaining increasing public prominence, countless volumes have been written on the proper care of the voice. It is therefore with some humility that I approach the task of discussing vocal hygiene.

---

*T*he best way to begin might be to consider the influence of the conditions that rule our daily lives. The most outstanding of these are probably *weather* and *climate*. By weather, I mean the daily changes and fluctuations of atmospheric conditions, while climate applies to the average weather in a given locale. Both weather and climate act primarily upon the surface of our body, the outer surface of the skin, and the hidden surface of the mucous membranes.

Among the mammals that require a stable body temperature for the maintenance of life, we humans rely most heavily on the skin as a regulator of body temperature. Exposed to high temperatures, our skin gives off body heat by perspiring, while in cold weather it helps preserve warmth through the constricting action of the fine blood capillaries. The vocal organs, too, are part of this balancing mechanism. As we saw in Chapter I, our noses bring inhaled air to the degree of temperature and humidity which the mucous membranes of the deeper respiratory tract require for good health.

With few exceptions, our North American climate is characterized by strong variations in temperature and humidity. It is somewhat paradoxical that the weather we like least is the best for our vocal organs and vice versa. On muggy days the air we inhale is warm and saturated with moisture, almost ideal for our mucous membranes. During a humid summer heat wave, of course, the boon to respiration is more than offset by the languishing effect of the weather on the body as a whole. But the nice crisp winter days with bright skies and invigorating winds are the dangerous ones. The incidence of respiratory infections reaches its peak not during the rainy period when everyone complains about the weather, but during cold spells when we are in high spirits and little inclined to worry about it. Then our nose finds it hard to keep up with the need for air conditioning, and our skin is chilled by icy winds. It is in such weather that our mucous membranes deserve special consideration. When we leave the house and walk along the street on a cold day carrying on a conversation, we are exposing our throat and vocal folds to the rigors of chilly dry air and depriving our mucous membrances of the warmth and moisture which only nose breathing can provide.

If you are in good physical condition, your body will not find it too difficult to adjust to the daily changes of the weather. People who work in the same place all year round do not ordinarily need to worry so much about the effect of atmospheric conditions on their vocal organs. Artists and lecturers, on the other hand, are faced with a different situation. Modern means of travel enable actors and actresses on the road, concert singers on tour, and lecturers whose itineraries call for appearances in a different city every night to move from one climatic zone to another quickly and abruptly.

The ease with which we can cross the continent, or even circle the earth, makes us forget the fact that our body is called upon to make tremendous adjustments. Our heart, blood vessels, lungs, skin, and mucous membranes are all sorely taxed while we are carried, within just a few hours, from the seacoast to the mountains, from temperate zones to the tropics. An artist who travels frequently has to be in good physical condition to stand the strain of such sudden adaptations. And even then you should, if at all possible, arrange your schedule to include a day of acclimatization before an appearance. If you have ever flown from the East Coast to Denver, for example, you will remember how dry and papery your throat felt after a few hours in the thin mountain air, how your heart beat faster, and your breathing was accelerated. In such a state, satisfactory voice performance is very difficult. Even intonation may suffer at high altitudes until the fine muscles which control the vocal folds have become adjusted to the low density of the air.

A horse, brought up from the plains to the mountains, refuses to canter until it has become acclimated. Human lungs, hearts and mucous membranes are entitled to the same consideration. Of course, humans have one big advantage over animals. We have learned to wear clothing as protection against the vicissitudes of the weather. The only trouble is that, to a large extent, clothing has lost its original purpose. It has become a symbol of social standing, a playground for constantly changing fashions, and has spoiled our natural powers of body resistance. From a strictly medical viewpoint, women often wear too little clothing and men too much. Women dress very sensibly in warm weather, but how they manage to brave winter days in cobweb stockings, open shoes, and hardly any underwear is a secret which a doctor cannot hope to understand. Men, on the other hand, insist on wearing numerous layers of clothing, shirts with closed collars, strangling neckties, and tight belts. But I do not expect to conquer the tyranny of fashion and convention by printed advice and, therefore, shall limit myself to a few remarks about the importance of proper clothing in the care of the vocal organs.

Apart from moral, esthetic, and social considerations, clothing has just one function: to form an insulating layer of air, under fabric, around the body. More harm is done by too many and too heavy clothes than by too few and too light ones. On the whole, healthy skin makes all the necessary adjustments with great speed, and light clothing keeps it in good condition. Dressing heavily to avoid colds quite frequently has the opposite effect.

One of my habitual patients is a middle-aged singer who comes to my office swaddled in every conceivable kind of garment. Watching him get undressed for a chest examination is to witness a major production. Having shed several mufflers, a heavy suit, a vest, and sweater, he finally emerges in long woolen underwear quite suitable for a Canadian fur trapper, which he does not shed until the first summer heat wave. In winter and summer, his skin lives in a permanent Turkish bath. Exhausted by so much sweating, it has long ceased to function as the body's main line of defense, and the result is a patient with an almost uninterrupted series of upper respiratory infections.

The case just cited may be an extreme one, but all too many singers still pamper their bodies by dressing too warmly. The younger generation is getting to be more sensible; light, informal clothing is definitely a boon to preservation of health and prevention of colds.

---

*P*roper *heating and air conditioning* of our homes and work places is another important factor in maintaining health. A good heating system should provide just enough warmth to make us feel comfortable, keep our heads cool and our feet warm, and at the same time, stabilize the humidity at a favorable level. Unfortunately, conventional heating meets none of these requirements. American homes, offices, and community buildings are notoriously overheated; the floors often are the coldest part of our rooms, and the already dry winter air is further dessicated by heating systems that dry out the air even more. European visitors keep asking us how we can stand it. The answer should be, we cannot.

Every fall, the beginning of the heating season brings to my offices singers, actors, and others who use their voices professionally, all complaining of dryness of the throat. Since we cannot easily change the heating system, the only way out is artificial humidification. This is easier said than done, however, for even when all windows and doors are closed, the air in a room is constantly changing. To keep it from becoming overly dry, moisture has to be added all the time. Relatively inexpensive humidifiers will bring relief to those suffering from dryness of the mucous membranes in the nose, throat, and larynx. In apartments and houses where the bedroom adjoins the bathroom, a humidifier can be improvised by leaving the door open and letting the hot shower run for a while.

Let us now consider the problem of *ventilation*. Whether or not to turn on the air conditioning or open the windows is an unresolved controversy between the advocates of tough living on one side and the enemies of draft on the other. Being inclined to sympathize with the fresh-air fans, I would like to report that, from a medical point of view, they are better equipped in the fight against colds. Actually, large-scale statistical research has shown no appreciable difference in the incidence of colds among those who sleep with windows open and those who do not.

The rule of common sense applies to ventilation just as it applies to the other subjects brought up in this discussion. There is a healthy medium between the singer who is forever concerned about catching a breath of cool air and the advocate of rigorous living who refuses to close the window in any weather. In the daytime when we are on the move, a healthy body can well endure a lot of fresh air; but when we are asleep, all body functions slow down and our skin and mucous membranes fare best when the temperature of the surrounding air is comfortable and even.

In the realm of personal habits, *nutrition* is an area in which the most serious offenses are committed. In this age of preoccupation with diets, almost all of us know exactly what foods we ought to eat and, it would appear, avoid them conscientiously. Many of us are forever overeating after having carefully selected the wrong things. We prefer the whitest of breads, the richest desserts, and still believe that meat is the most important food.

There does not seem to be much sense in repeating what you can read in almost every magazine, namely, that our diet should be well planned, with a strong accent on fresh vegetables fruit, and whole grains. Everybody knows that anyhow. The spirit is strong, but the sweet tooth is our weakness. Let me only point out that the mucous membranes prefer a diet in which starches and dairy products are limited to a minimum. This is especially important in those cases in which an overproduction of phlegm interferes with free nasal breathing and clarity of the voice.

Overindulgence in starches and sugars is, of course, mainly responsible for making us a nation with a tendency to overweight. Conversely, public taste demands that the artists who appear in public be thin. The fat singer is a thing of the past. As a result, countless performers are forever struggling to keep their weight down to a minimum, frequently to the detriment of general and vocal health.

Everyone has an optimum weight which best suits his or her body structure. Generally speaking, that weight is somewhat less than what most men over forty actually weigh, and somewhat more than what most women of all ages consider desirable. Rather than alternating between sporadic spells of rapid reducing when the newest nine-day wonder diet appears in your favorite newspaper and subsequent flings of overeating, it is far wiser to maintain one's body weight at the level which experience has shown to be most conducive to the maintenance of well-being, vigor and resistance.

Just a word about the timing of meals. Almost everyone who performs in public instinctively avoids eating a heavy meal before an appearance. Afterwards, however, there is the temptation to eat too much. The release of tensions after a performance brings with it proverbial hunger and thirst, which easily leads to overindulgence in food and drink at very late hours. Poor sleep and overweight are usually the result.

We all have become very *vitamin* conscious in recent years and help support a gigantic industry that produces the multicolored capsules, which we take to atone for all dietary transgressions. Actually, a well-planned diet contains all necessary vitamins in sufficient amounts. If you eat properly, you should not need vitamin pills.

Still, it cannot be denied that a surprisingly large number of people — rich as well as poor — have borderline cases of vitamin deficiency. Many of these deficiencies manifest themselves in the mucous membranes of the respiratory tract. It is, therefore, quite important to watch the professional vocalist for possible signs of vitamin shortage.

In taking vitamins, one fact must be kept in mind: the body does not store vitamins but accepts them only in the amounts that are needed at a given time. In other words, if you buy and take vitamins with which your body is already amply supplied, you are throwing your money away. Do not shop around for bargains when purchasing vitamins. An inexpensive brand might well be useless because the amount of vitamins is too small, because prolonged storage has led to deterioration in the capsule, or worse, but fortunately not infrequently, because an irresponsible manufacturer has misstated the actual contents.

It is with some hesitation that I approach our next subject — the use of nicotine and alcohol. We are all given daily updates on the ever-expanding list of harmful, often fatal, effects of smoking and drinking, both personally and societally. I propose to limit my discussion to an evaluation of both substances as they affect the vocal organs.

The case against *nicotine* is simple. We are not concerned here with its proven toxic effects on the heart and the blood vessels, but rather with the direct irritation of the mucous membranes caused by the inhaled smoke. In this respect, pipe and cigar smoking is somewhat less harmful since deep inhalation is rarely practiced, although recent studies of the effects of "second-hand smoke" do indicate that inhalation of smoke-laden air in any quantity may be very harmful in the long run. However, the cigarette smoker who brings the smoke down to the vocal folds, windpipe, and bronchi is the real and immediate sufferer. Whenever I want to demonstrate the effect of smoking to a recalcitrant patient, I perform a little experiment which you can easily repeat for your own enlightenment. Blow cigarette smoke into a highball glass, cover the glass with a sheet of white paper, turn it upside down, and let it stand for a few minutes. You will then see a distinct yellow circle — it shows up better in daylight — and you will realize the extent of irritation of your mucous membranes by the continuous deposits of coal tars from the smoke.

For thousands of years, alcohol has been used because of its stimulating, or rather inhibition-loosening, effect on the brain. If taken before a performance to overcome the tensions of stage fright, its blessings are questionable. Alcohol interferes with judgment, substituting a delusive satisfaction for real mastery of performance, and it impairs muscular coordination and physical efficiency to an extent which might well be deterimental to the speaker or singer. Besides, alcohol dilates the blood capillaries and thus causes an increased production of mucus — an added undesirable effect on the vocal organs.

Habitual use of alcohol is definitely harmful to the voice as the rough hoarseness of the "whiskey tenor" will attest. Finally, alcohol upsets the delicate heat balance of the body. It gives our skin a deceptive feeling of warmth, while we are losing heat at a rapid rate. Such chilling makes the body more vulnerable to colds. As long as you limit your consumption of alcohol to an occasional drink *following* a performance and avoid exposure to cold weather afterward, no harm is done.

By now you are undoubtedly tired of being told what not to do and having *Verboten* signs plastered all over your personal life. So, for a change, let us turn to the things you *can* and should do.

Rest, for instance. Although we often complain that the mad rush of modern life does not give us sufficient time for rest, we all agree that plenty of sleep at night and refreshing siestas during the day are highly desirable. I dislike intensely giving commonplace advice, which is easily pronounced but hard to follow (such as the doctor's famous stand-by, "take it easy for a while"). The competitive struggle for professional success usually leaves most of us little latitude in shaping personal habits. Yet it must be said that a fair amount of undisturbed sleep is essential to the maintenance of good general health and for proper functioning and resilience of the vocal organs. In this connection, singers are often confronted with a special problem: how to get the necessary rest before a vocal performance.

When it comes to international travel, the changing of times zones puts the body under additional stress. The inner clock that runs our physical balance is upset. I always advise artists who have to cross the Atlantic, and even more the Pacific, to spend a full day after arrival at their hotel before they officially "arrive" to give the body a chance to acclimatize.

The curse of traveling lecturers, actors and actresses, and singers on the road is the pressure of social obligations. They are often asked to accept well-meant invitations to luncheons, teas, and receptions. Even at the risk of incurring the displeasure of hostesses and agents, it is far wiser to decline such voice-straining engagements politely and to rest up for the evening's performance instead.

---

*W*ith certain reservations, regular moderate exercise is healthy and can be heartily endorsed. By moderate, I mean not only the amount of exercise, but also the spirit in which it is undertaken. Voice professionals of all types work under considerable nervous strain. Exercise should help them to relax and take their mind off their worries, but competitive games only add new tensions. We can learn a lesson from the protagonists of real sportsmanship, the old Greeks and the English, who have never forgotten that sport is basically play. The often-heard expression "to play hard" is a contradiction in itself.

If you are middle-aged and not accustomed to regular exercise, do not decide that now is the time to recapture your youthful figure through strenuous athletics. The consequences might be disastrous. Start easily and slowly. Swimming is an ideal sport for the vocalist. It stimulates the skin and encourages deep breathing and smooth muscle action. Walking, also, is one of the best forms of exercise. Jogging is excellent for younger people and others in good physical condition since it improves control and economy of breathing. However, from a medical point of view, the value of golf lies mainly in the fact that it induces people to walk a couple of miles.

Whatever form of exercise you prefer, do it at a leisurely pace, forget about scores, and, above all, enjoy yourself.

*E*ver since the famous English throat specialist Morel Mackenzie — who, by the way, wrote in 1888 the first scientific book on the hygiene of the vocal organs, which is still a classic — published his observations on the connection between the female reproductive organs and the nasal turbinates, we have known that many women suffer from nasal congestion immediately before and at the beginning of their menstrual periods. We have, furthermore, learned to regard the whole respiratory tract as a unit that is sensitive to changes in the hormonal balance. Many women experience no discomfort in the nose or lower respiratory tract during menstruation, but others do in varying degrees. A number of women also develop abdominal discomfort that interferes with free breathing, and many women suffer from various physical and emotional problems caused by the Premenstrual Syndrome (PMS).

As a general rule, singing or acting during menstruation will have no harmful effects as long as the artist does not try to overcome any indisposition by force. Here again, superior technique is the surest compensation for any temporary impairment of perfect vocal function. Do not expect to be at your best during the menstrual period, avoid, if possible, important engagements which produce additional tensions, and rely on your technique. But do not use any force which might harm your voice.

European opera companies have a special clause in their contracts which permits female singers to excuse themselves from all performances during the menstrual period. Schedules are filed with the management and plans made accordingly. In the United States, on the other hand, artists are expected to and do perform without regard to menstruation.

Pregnancy interferes rarely with voice performance during the first five or six months. Some women are able to sing freely and without effort up to an advanced stage of pregnancy. Generally, however, it is best to avoid professional singing and acting during the last months. Not only may hormonal influences on the mucous membranes become more pronounced at that time, but the growth of the baby may interfere with abdominal breathing.

After delivery, the overstretched abdominal muscles slowly return to their normal state. In view of the importance of abdominal breathing and muscular control for vocal quality, special care must be taken to strengthen the abdominal muscles. Breathing exercises should be resumed very soon, followed by active muscular training and moderate vocalization, assuming there are no medical problems that would prevent this.

*A*llergy of any marked degree constitutes a handicap for the speaker or singer and requires care and treatment. The majority of all allergies are due to substances we inhale — like pollen, dust, animal hair, and molds — and produce respiratory symptoms such as congestion of the nose, sneezing, running discharge, itching of the throat, cough, and wheezing from the chest. At the peak of an allergic attack or during a seasonal bout, as with hay fever, the normal functioning of the vocal organs is impaired, sometimes to the extent of total professional disability.

Seasonally limited allergies are bad enough. Ragweed hay fever, for instance (from which literally millions of people suffer in the United States), lasts until the end of September and makes the opening of the music and theatrical season pure torment for many artists. Dust and other year-round allergies are even worse, in that they constantly interfere with professional activities. Above all, an untreated allergy may lead to asthmatic symptoms, one of the severest handicaps under which a speaker or vocal artist can labor.

For these reasons, *treatment* of an allergy is part of vocal hygiene. Limitations of space forbid going into details. You will need the help of a medical professional with special experience in testing and treating allergic conditions. Suffice it to say that allergies — once determined by conclusive tests — can be dealt with in three ways: by eliminating the offending agents, by building up resistance through so-called desensitization, or by the use of drugs.

Elimination of the offending agent by excluding such foods from the diet is possible in cases of food allergies. To a lesser extent, it is feasible with animal hair and dust. Household pets can be banished, and pillows and mattresses can be protected with dustproof covers. Air conditioning affords temporary relief, but the patient feels worse after leaving the comfort of filtered air.

Antihistamines do *not* cure allergy. They only suppress symptoms. They are valuable in providing fast, temporary relief, but they do not create any resistance to allergy. Besides, these drugs produce unwanted secondary effects, such as drowsiness which interferes with the presence of mind, reliability of memory and muscular coordination so important to the speaker, actor and singer, in a large percentage of patients. Furthermore, the purely symptomatic action of antihistamines gives no protection against the danger of developing asthmatic troubles.

In attempting to control allergies, our best bet is still *desensitization* — the gradual building up of resistance by injections of allergen extracts of increasing strength. This method produces excellent results in cases of pollen and dust allergies, especially if combined with occasional small doses of antihistamines on peak days of exposure.

Treatment of allergy is one aspect of vocal hygiene which definitely calls for professional medical help, which may mean the difference between an insurmountable handicap in the professional use of the voice and a wide margin of safety and freedom from discomfort.

Artists who depend on the free function of their vocal organs have a tendency to develop dependency on medications that may be, at best, superfluous and at worst dangerous. I would like to mention two such abuses. Cortisone in very small doses for just a few days could be used by your laryngologist to restore a clear voice after a bout of acute laryngitis, but it is not a drug that should be used frequently and without strict supervision. Singers who travel professionally a great deal and who have experienced at home the benefit derived from such medication may ask the physician they see abroad to prescribe it again when they do not feel up to par. Used often, cortisone can become a risky habit that should be avoided.

More recently, a number of prescription and illegal drugs have become fashionable for fighting stage fright and increasing self-confidence. I am very much against such use. To some degree, anxiety before an important performance is a natural phenomenon. Many famous artists experience it constantly, but they learn to live with it. Stage fright is the building up of tensions that is necessary for the creative process of the artistic performance, which erupts in a blaze of artistic mastery once the curtain goes up, and it should not be fought. To depend on the use of a drug interferes with the artistic secret and

creates a dangerous addiction. Still, stage fright is the curse of the performing artist. In some instances it can wreck a career, and it may
require the help of a psychotherapist.

*F*rom birth until death, our voices reflect the various stages of
physical development through which we pass. The first cry of the
baby, the child's high-pitched voice, the changing voice of the adolescent, all play an important part toward the final shaping of the adult
speaking and singing voice.

Very little is known about the influence of advanced age on the
vocal organs. This is particularly regrettable when we consider that
with rising life expectancy the number of older people is on the
increase and includes many who use their voice professionally such as
teachers, ministers, lawyers, and even singers.

Geriatrics, the science dealing with the diseases of the aged,
should attract the interest of all those who specialize in speech and
voice therapy. Study of the effects of hormonal, vitamin, drug, and
exercise therapy on the aging voice may result in a more active
approach to the problem. Until such time, I must restrict myself to
describing the effects of advancing age on the voice. The joints between the cartilages of the larynx move less smoothly; the cartilages
themselves become more rigid; muscle coordination is impaired; and
muscular strength is weakened. This results in the loss of vocal power,
uncertainty of intonation, and the typical tremolo and wavering we
associate with older people's voices. Changes in the hormonal balance
may cause inversion of the sex characteristic — the male voice becoming higher and the female voice assuming a masculine timbre. As with
all of the other bodily changes which accompany old age, wide individual differences exist with regard to the rapidity and intensity of
such changes. Constitutional and hereditary factors have a determining influence, and it is at this point also that the long-term effects of a
well-regulated life make themselves felt.

The professional speaker will find it much easier to adjust to
advancing age than the singer, who may feel the negative effects
much sooner. It was indeed an unforgettable experience to have heard
the great Mattia Battistini sing *Don Giovanni* at the age of seventy.
But many others age prematurely in voice as well as in body. Those
with poor vocal technique are the first to fall by the wayside, while a
singer who has devoted a lifetime to perfecting his technique and preserving health intelligently may be able to lead an active professional
life in spite of advancing years.

It is indeed hard for the artist who is young in spirit and rich in accumulated experience to accept the inevitability of age. One of the saddest aspects of a voice doctor's practice is to witness the decline of a great voice after the age of sixty and to have to watch the hopeless struggle of many artists who try, often in the face of financial insecurity, to prolong a career which is rapidly coming to an end.

The only thing that may ease this situation is to help the artist face the facts and come to terms with reality. Here, as is so frequently the case, the doctor's task is mainly a psychological one; but it is a frustrating experience which makes us hope that further research will equip us to take a more active approach.

*T*his chapter has become rather long, as was to be expected, since I have dealt with a key subject in our field. Eight out of ten questions which are addressed to me after a lecture on voice problems concern the hygiene of everyday living. As we have said in the beginning, when it comes to hygiene of the vocal organs, the advice of old Quintilian and the teachers of Italian Bel Canto is hard to beat: Keep your body in good shape to withstand the rigors of wind and weather, dress sensibly but do not undermine your resistance by pampering yourself, plan your meals in accordance with nutritional requirements, get as much rest and sleep as possible, and exercise moderately.

Finding the proper middle course between the two equally dangerous extremes of willfully neglecting the body and oversolicitous pampering is the most important maxim in vocal hygiene. As long as the body and the vocal organs are accustomed to a healthy routine, an occasional fling will do no harm. As in all other areas of life, common sense is what matters.

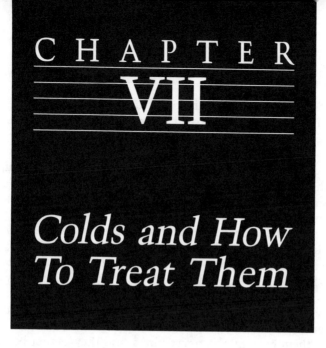

CHAPTER VII

Colds and How To Treat Them

Sooner or later, everbody gets a cold. Some of us might be lucky and escape colds for a while because of high personal resistance or lack of infecting contacts. The average person keeps getting colds with depressing regularity, at least twice a year. Colds, as has been said very often, are inescapable as weather, death, and taxes. And contrary to popular opinion, not even the climate you live in makes much difference. If you do not rely on the claims of chambers of commerce but on "cold" statistics, you will find almost the same rate of infection in Florida, the Midwest, Southern California, and Alaska.

This is as it should be, because the common cold is first and foremost an *infection*. As a rule, people are strangely reluctant to accept this fact. Their attitude is a classic example of the influence of a semantic error on our thinking. The term "cold" has stressed the part played by chilling in contracting a cold to the degree that the importance of infection is always underrated. Consequently, people with colds feel often compelled to search for some "mistake" they must have made. Mumps and measles are accepted as unavoidable accidents, because we know that infection can hit us when we expect it least. But we react to colds as if we had committed a sin. We search our conscience for the window we forgot to close, the muffler we left behind, the rubbers we should have worn.

True, chilling plays a part in the mechanism of getting a cold, but it is not the decisive factor. You may become the victim of a cold without any chilling but *never* without an infection with the virus of the common cold.

We hear a lot about *viruses* these days. What used to be an interesting research problem known only to bacteriologists has become a household word. "Viral infection" is now a convenient label for all kinds of fevers of unknown origin. Viruses are different from bacteria in a number of negative ways. They cannot be seen under an ordinary microscope (except as bare shadows with tremendous electronic enlargement), they cannot be separated from any fluid that contains them even by the finest filters, and they cannot be isolated and cultured by the usual laboratory methods.

The list of infectious diseases that are caused by viruses is very long. Measles, German measles, mumps, polio, influenza, and now AIDS, to mention only a few, are viral infections.

The *virus of the common cold* beats them all in omnipresence and frequency of infection. The cold virus is unique in that it acts as the door-opener for many bacterial infections. The virus attacks first, weakens the resistance of the mucous membranes which then may be invaded by germs — like streptococci, staphylococci, and pneumococci — that lurk everywhere. If they take over, all kinds of complications may develop, such as ear infections, sinusitis, tonsillitis, laryngitis, bronchitis, and pneumonia. If it remains limited to the primary cold virus infection, the common cold is a relatively harmless, self-limited disease. Its significance and importance lie in the possibility of secondary bacterial infections. Most virus infections leave in their wake a longlasting immunity, some — like measles — for life, others for years. But a cold can hit again after only a short time. This is because the cold virus is not a single unchanging agent but a whole family including perhaps hundreds of different viruses. Like the virus of influenza, it changes constantly, with new and different strains appearing often.

Chilling diminishes the resistance of our mucous membranes to infection. It has to be rather protracted to lower the temperature of the nasal surfaces by contraction of the small blood vessels. The draft from an open window, the blast of the wind at the street corner are, as a rule, offset by the ability of our body to make fast adjustments to changes in temperature.

We get a cold because somebody gives the virus to us and because our resistance to infection has dropped to a low level. We look at every open window with fear, but we weaken our body resistance by lack of sleep, poor eating habits, and the hectic rush of modern life.

There is no need to describe the symptoms of a cold. We all know them from frequent experience. While to the average person an uncomplicated cold is just a nuisance to be borne with more or less grace, it is the terror of the man or woman who uses his or her voice professionally. To them, colds constitute an ever present occupational hazard. The battlefield of the cold and of its complications are the vocal organs. The cold impairs their function, usually at the most inopportune moments. The cold leads the list of the pet hates of singers, actors and actresses or speakers, even ahead of critics, producers or unreceptive audiences.

Unfortunately, no specific therapy exists against the common cold. As long as no drug that attacks the virus of the cold is available, the defense against the invader is left to the powers of resistance of the body. The only sensible treatment of colds consists of making it easier for the body to concentrate on the job of fighting the infection by relieving it, as much as possible, from other work. In other words, taking the cold seriously, staying at home or, even better, in bed for a day or two. But that goes against human nature. We all talk about our colds, we annoy our families by complaining about our misery, we want to be pitied as a patient, but we refuse to behave like one. We keep on running around, spreading infection right and left; and, instead of giving our body a fair chance, we "treat" our cold with our favorite remedies.

In treating colds, everybody is an expert. There is no other field in medicine where superstitions, time-honored misconceptions, and short-lived fads are so widely practiced and hotly defended as in dealing with a cold. One of the oldest favorites with cold patients is alcohol. People are seldom at loss for an excuse to take a drink, but in the case of an approaching cold, the belief in the germ-killing abilities of alcohol gives a special medical dignity to the consumption of a few drinks. Actually, alcohol fights infection only if rubbed on the skin. Taken internally, it upsets the heat balance of the body. It dilates the blood vessels and gives us a deceptive feeling of warmth. The skin loses heat rapidly while we feel comfortable.

The patient who takes a drink to fight the chilliness of the first stage of a cold and then proceeds with daily chores only creates more favorable conditions for intense chilling without becoming aware of it. No amount of alcohol will disturb the cold virus in its temporary conquest of the body.

If you begin to sneeze, your first reflex is probably to open the drawer or the medicine chest where you keep your favorite brand of tablets for just this emergency. Thanks to tremendous advertising, aspirin is your most likely choice. Again I have to disappoint you by saying that aspirin has no direct effect whatsoever on the cold virus. Aspirin is another name for acetylsalicylic acid. It belongs to the family of the so-called antipyretics. They inhibit the heat regulating centers of the brain and, to a certain degree, lower body temperatures by perspiration. An increase in temperature is one of the devices the body uses to fight infection. To bring the temperature of the blood down makes us feel more comfortable but, at the same time, counteracts the self-help of nature.

Aspirin and related drugs like acetaminophen, available in dozens of combinations under as many different brand names, have their place in medicine as mild pain killers. Some of the complications of the common cold create pain. These drugs are then helpful to take the edge off the discomfort until the infection is conquered. But in the fight against the cold, they are without value.

If we cannot fight a cold actively, we can, at least, try to alleviate the symptoms as much as possible. Of these, the stuffiness of the nose and the profuse nasal discharge are particularly unpleasant. For relief of nasal blockage nose drops are widely used. The ideal *nose sprays* should contain a *vasoconstrictor,* one of the drugs which make the nasal membranes shrink by contraction of the small blood vessels; they should be *isotonic,* meaning equal in concentration to the body fluids; and they should be slightly *alkaline.*

The most widely used vasoconstrictor is *ephedrine,* which produces a mild shrinking of the mucous membranes. It is available under a variety of brand names. They all use a watery basis of isotonic concentration. The simplest isotonic diluent is saline, a .9 percent solution of salt in distilled water which equals the concentration of salt in the body fluids.

Alkalinity of nose drops is desirable because the important self-cleaning mechanism of the mucous membranes by ciliary action (see Chapter II) depends on the slight alkalinity of the nasal mucus. In colds and other infections, the nose becomes slightly acid, which results in a slowing down or stopping of ciliary movement. Slightly alkaline medication helps to restore normal ciliary function and ephedrine in saline fulfills this need.

The nose sprays that can be bought at any drug store produce a fine spray that covers the surfaces of the nasal cavities. A puff of it in each of the nostrils is sufficient to produce better ventilation. Used too often and for more than a few days, the negative effect of nasal congestion after the beneficial shrinking of the nasal membranes has worn off becomes more pronounced. Worse, you can become physically or psychologically dependent upon the relief the sprays provide.

When using these nose sprays try to avoid contact of tip of the bottle with the nostril. It happens easily and leads to a contamination of the sterile contents of the bottle. Bottles with nose sprays should *never* be used again for another cold or by another person. The contents are almost invariably polluted with hosts of germs.

Even if it hurts you, throw your nose sprays into the garbage can when your cold is gone. The half-filled bottle you like to save for future use will cost you dearly by giving you or your family "nose spray disease" a few months later.

A certain amount of congestion of the mucuous membranes and of nasal discharge is quite desirable. It brings the healing forces of the blood into the infected area and helps to throw off the invading germs and the debris of the battle. Overdosage of vasoconstrictors will only prolong the normal course of a cold.

Modern medicine has opened so many new avenues for active approach in the treatment of diseases that we have, somehow, lost sight of the fact that the main burden in conquering infection will always be with the body. Give it rest from all unnecessary work, and it will expel the cold virus within a few days. The professional speaker or singer stands to lose more by the complications of colds that are the inevitable result of running around with an infection. Ounces of nose drops and bottles of tablets will not do for you what one day in the equalizing warmth of your bed can achieve.

Local heat is one of the oldest remedies for all kinds of local aches. To expose an infected part of our body to any form of local heat means to create hyperemia, an increased flood of healing blood through the dilated blood vessels of skin or deeper tissues. The short-wave or diathermy machines which lend so much glamour to the doctor's office are needed where deeper parts of the body have to be reached by radiating heat.

To get heat to the mucous membranes of nose and throat, the old-fashioned inhalation of steam serves just as well. If you use it at home, you have to keep two points in mind. The dilation of blood vessels, which is the immediate consequence of the application of local heat, might increase the discomfort in your already congested nose. If that happens you are better off without it. Also, do not inhale steam if you have to leave the house shortly afterward. During a cold the mucous membranes have temporarily lost their ability to make quick adjustments to changes in temperature. To wake up in the morning with a cold, swallow a couple of aspirins, inhale steam for five minutes, dry your face while you gulp your coffee, and then rush out to work is to court disaster. The aspirin will make you perspire, thereby cooling the skin; the overheated mucous membranes will be chilled by the cold outside air; the germs that lie in wait will have a field day. You will return in the evening with the makings of a fine sinusitis, laryngitis, or even bronchitis.

So far I have spoken only of the effects of a cold on the nose. The professional speaker or singer will worry almost as much or even more about the throat. Many colds begin with a tickling or burning sensation in the upper part of the throat. Too many professionals have the habit of constantly "treating" their throat with all kinds of medication, by way of gargles and medicated lozenges. In times of colds, they redouble their efforts in the mistaken belief that they can kill the infection by such measures. However, the disinfectants in gargles must be extremely diluted to suit our mucous membranes. Gargling brings them in contact with the throat for a few seconds. How can one expect any germ-killing effect from so short and so weak a contact? The only good that can come from gargling is a superficial kind of cleaning. If the gargle is at least hot, it helps to attract the blood into the irritated throat and to stimulate a soothing flow of mucus. Whether you apply local heat by steam, hot gargles, or hot drinks, it is always the temporary hyperemia that relieves your throat, not the effect of any drugs or special foods you may add to them.

The case for *lozenges* rests on a rather doubtful basis too. Lozenge is a French intruder into the English language, reminding us of past centuries when fashionable people who had never heard of a toothbrush sucked perfumed pastilles for obvious reasons. The lozenges and cough drops that are sold to the public by the millions have little effect on the throat. The drugs they contain are weak and without therapeutic value. The glycerine that forms the base of many lozenges dries out the membranes because of its hydroscopic (water-binding) action. The best that can be said about lozenges is that they stimulate the flow of saliva by the movements of the tongue.

The constant habit of many singers and speakers of using lozenges whenever the throat feels dry confuses the effect of nervous tensions on the throat with the infectious irritation of the cold. The sucking of a lozenge before a speech or an appearance is a kind of psychotherapeutic self-treatment that is, at least, more harmless than a cigarette or a drink.

Aromatic compounds have been used in all forms for thousands of years. Camphor, menthol, and aromatic oils (like eucalyptus, pine needle, and turpentine) were already great favorites in the Greek and Roman eras, and they are still dear to the hearts of cold-suffering patients. They are soothing to mucous membranes because they create a sensation of coolness. In the nose, they are irritating and should not be used. In sprays and lozenges for the throat, they do no harm and satisfy the desire of the patients for a comforting sickroom odor that gives their troubles a certain distinction.

Oral cold vaccines — taken by mouth in tablet or capsule form — have, so far, produced very unsatisfactory results. All research workers who have tested them on large groups agree in rejecting these vaccines. The only type of vaccination that has proven at all effective is the use of influenza vaccines. The vaccine, however, affords protection only against the most common strains of influenza virus.

When antihistamines were first introduced with loud fanfares in the press, massive advertising, and tremendous sales, hope was high that they were the answer to the common cold. Since then, the medical professional has had the opportunity to evaluate these drugs, and, just as the experts predicted, the results are disappointing indeed. Colds are infections. Antihistamines are drugs that suppress allergic symptoms, but they do not cure or prevent colds.

Altogether, I have to admit that no active therapy of any kind will influence the short course of a common cold with any degree of efficiency. You might now, with some justification, object to the title of this chapter as a promise that was not kept. But I have to remind you again that one effective self-treatment of colds exists: rest, rest the body in its fight against the infection and rest the vocal organs which cannot stand the double burden of local warfare against the invader and of highly complex function in professional use.

There is no better way of *preventing a cold* than to build up a healthy body. It is impossible to avoid exposure, especially in wintertime when most everyone sneezes and coughs at us. But it is possible to increase resistance. A body whose resistance has been undermined by inadequate diet, too much heavy clothing, and too little rest and exercise is easily conquered by infection. Therefore, everything we do to build up the body's strength, resilience, and hardiness helps to protect us against respiratory infections.

There is no shortcut to good health. You cannot prevent colds by simply taking pills. The common cold is a virus infection which produces only a short-lived immunity and as yet no effective vaccine exists.

To Voltaire is ascribed the malicious remark that "medicine is the art of entertaining the patient while nature takes care of the healing." As wrong as this witticism might be in many medical emergencies that require energetic action, it serves to remind us that, in most diseases, it is the body itself that does the actual healing.

Somehow it goes against the grain of our hyperactive Western philosophy of life to deal with an unpleasant situation in a passive way. Even in minor diseases, like a cold, we feel compelled to do something about it. If you follow Voltaire, your only self-treatment of your next cold should consist of entertaining yourself while nature takes care of the rest. You might watch television, solve a crossword puzzle or read a book — maybe even this one — but otherwise just make it easy for your body to do the healing. Stay home for a day, preferably in bed, eat lightly, and keep your bowels open — without resorting to harsh drugs. Blow your nose gently to avoid pressing infected mucus into sinuses or middle ears. Use nose sprays sparingly to reduce nasal congestion. If you have a headache, take aspirin, no more than three or four during the day.

With this regime, your cold will soon be over, without requiring the help of a doctor. The sacrifice of a day or two at home will pay good dividends in fast recovery or in avoidance of complications. A normal common cold should be broken in four to six days. If, in spite of reasonable precautions, no improvement of the condition should be observed within this time, it will be necessary to seek medical advice.

Other complications that require medical advice are:

- The development of laryngitis. This frequent and usually harmless sequel of a cold is, of course, a great handicap for the speaker and singer and requires special treatment.
- Severe headaches or localized pain, which might indicate a complication in sinuses, tonsils, ears.
- Fever that exceeds the mild increase in body temperature we have to expect in the beginning of a cold. Any oral temperature above 99.4 degrees is real fever, indicating a complicating secondary infection.
- Cough, which follows the downward development of the infection into the deeper respiratory tract.

I will devote a special chapter to these complications, but before doing so I should like to take you first on a conducted tour through the office of the doctor you are going to see. I shall try to explain to you the medical instruments, the methods of examination, and the route by which the physician arrives at a diagnosis.

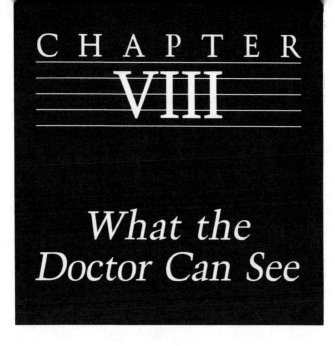

CHAPTER
VIII

What the Doctor Can See

Nobody, except a hypochondriac, likes to go to the doctor. The reasons for the visit — unless it is for a checkup — are already unpleasant — something is wrong in the body, one of the organs does not function properly, there is pain; our health, which we like to take for granted, seems to be threatened.

Patients waiting in the doctor's office — too often unnecessarily long — are worried. They fear a diagnosis that may confirm their apprehensions; they consider with misgivings the prospect of a prolonged treatment; and they dislike the necessity of having to spend good money on doctors and medicine.

In this uncomfortable situation, patients need and should receive encouragement and reassurance, which must come from the personality of the doctor. A few words of sympathy can go a long way in creating the confidence that one's body is in good hands. Still, faith in the doctor's ability and understanding does not remove all your apprehensions. Most patients do not cherish the idea of having to submit their bodies to the impersonal probing of a medical examination, to instruments, tests, and other methods quite outside of their ordinary experience.

In this respect, the examination of the ear, nose, throat, and larynx confronts the patients with a lot of mysterious instrumentation. Each step is done with artificial lighting and strange instruments, all in regions of the body that are hidden from sight and unknown to the average person.

A better understanding of the *technique of examination* is the best help in this situation. The patient who knows what to expect will feel much more at ease and will submit with better relaxation to an examination which requires good cooperation by the patient. For this reason I should like to pretend that you, the reader, have learned the secret of the famous "invisible man." Quietly and unseen, you sit in the corner of the examination room of a laryngologist to observe the doctor at work. I will remain at your side — authors are invisible anyhow — to explain to you what you see.

The room you find yourself in has the usual aseptic and utilitarian look of all such places. What distinguishes it from, for instance, the family practitioner's examination room is the lack of the usual bright lights. The special problem in the examination of ear, nose, or throat is that deep recesses of the body have to be made visible by artificial illumination. A semidark room provides a better contrast to the lighting effect of a spotlight, furnished by the head mirror. To increase this effect, the walls may also be painted in the pale blues or greens that are used in operating rooms.

Near one wall stands a chair with head and armrests for the patient and a small stool for the doctor. On one side of the patient's chair, you find a lamp with a strong concentrated light. A table or cabinet exhibits the instruments for routine examination, bottles with different drugs, sprays, and containers for cotton and gauze. An electric pump provides air pressure for sprays and other gadgets and suction for a number of uses.

Now the doctor enters the room wearing the *head mirror.* Next to the syringe and stethoscope, the head mirror is probably the best known of all medical instruments. But its function is poorly understood, at least by most cartoonists who frequently draw it, to the dismay of the laryngologist, in a wrong position.

The invention of the head mirror solved the problem that confronted Manuel Garcia and the early medical investigators of the larynx: how to obtain sufficient shadow-free light for their observations. Garcia, as you might remember from the introduction, made his first observation of the vocal cords in sunlight. Dr. J. Czermak who experimented in Budapest with the new laryngeal mirror hit on the happy idea of using a concave (inward curved) mirror to concentrate light from a candle. In 1858 he constructed the first *head mirror*. Since then, it has been changed only in small constructional details.

Fixed to a headband by an adjustable clamp, the head mirror concentrates the light from a bulb into a powerful beam. The hole in the middle of the mirror permits the doctor to look along the axis of this beam. If you watch your doctor at work, you will see that before each examination he swings the mirror into position so that the hole is in front of one of his eyes. The light from the lamp at the side of the patient is caught in the mirror and reflected — as a small but very bright beam — to the face of the patient. During examination or treatment, the doctor has to hold his head absolutely still for steady illumination.

Now a patient is shown into the examination room. We are lucky because he is a young singer who has come in for a general checkup. His teacher had the good sense to tell him that a professional singer or speaker should pick his throat specialist in healthy days and ask for a thorough checkup of all vocal organs.

The doctor who has studied the patient's body under normal conditions and has observed, on various occasions, its reaction to infection, drugs, and treatments, is in a much better position to help than the once-consulted physician. The modern habit of changing doctors constantly, at the slightest displeasure or on the vaguest recommendation, does great disservice to the patient. True, there are valid reasons why a patient may want to and should change doctors. But the "floating" patient who never gives doctors a chance beyond a few treatments is, as a rule, as badly off as the vocal student who runs from one teacher to another one.

In the meantime, the doctor has finished the preliminary questioning of the patient and begins with the examination. First, the *ears* are looked into. A small, funnel-shaped instrument, called an ear speculum, is inserted into the ear canal while the auricle is pulled backward and upward. Thus, the s-shaped ear canal is straightened out, and the eardrum becomes visible.

Next comes the *nose*. With your knowledge of nasal anatomy, you realize the difficulty of examining the narrow cavities through the small openings of the nostrils. The doctor grasps the nasal speculum, an instrument with small blunt blades which are inserted into the nostrils and spread. The speculum keeps the hairs in the nostrils out of the way and widens the nostrils. To judge from the peaceful look in the patient's face it does not hurt at all.

Now, the doctor takes a spray bottle from the table, connects it with the pressure hose of the motor pump and directs a fine spray into the nostrils, then waits for a few minutes. If you think of our discussion of vasoconstrictors in the last chapter, you can guess the purpose of this procedure. Under the influence of the spray, the mucous membranes shrink and permit a better inspection of all the structures in the nose: the septum, the turbinates, and the meati. The middle meatus (see Chapter I) gets special attention because there most of the openings of the sinuses are found. Freedom of air passage — a necessity for proper function of the nose — is tested, and deviations of the septum from the ideal straight line are noted.

Few people, by the way, have a completely straight septum. Even marked *septum deviations* are not harmful in themselves. They are significant and require correction only if they hinder nasal ventilation or block drainage of the sinuses. The conservative approach that has replaced the surgical enthusiasm of earlier years has limited septum operations to a few strict indications.

The rest of the examination of our patient is done through the open *mouth.* Our patient — a new hand in such a situation — hastens to assure the doctor that no instrument would be necessary for an inspection of his throat. The doctor smiles, because this remark is common. Quite a few patients have an intense dislike of any instrumental manipulation in their throat, particularly the use of a tongue depressor. The reasons for this apprehension usually go back to childhood. It may be simply the memory of clumsy handling of a tongue depressor that was pushed with force into the throat of a struggling youngster. But sometimes the fear of oral examination emerges from deeper layers of our personality. As we now know, oral satisfaction or displeasure is an important factor in the emotional life of earliest childhood, and the adult resistance to oral examination is just one of the telltales that betray earlier conflicts.

Our doctor does not try to force the examination on the patient but explains that a satisfactory examination of the mouth and throat cannot be done without the help of some instruments, and that cooperation of the patient makes the examination easy for both doctor and patient. Finally, the doctor points out that a future singer — or any professional of the voice — will see a throat doctor more frequently than the average person. The sooner the patient learns to relax his tongue and throat, in spite of instrumental handling, the faster he will lose all apprehension in this situation.

Reassured, our patient submits to fate. He opens his mouth while the doctor presses his tongue gently down, out of the field of vision. The soft palate with the uvula and the tonsils — amazingly enough, a number of patients are lucky enough to still have them — and then the throat are inspected.

The *nasopharynx,* the space behind the soft palate, cannot be seen by direct observation. The doctor takes a small circular mirror attached to a long handle, warms it over a flame, and then holds it (without touching the throat) behind the soft palate. By turning it slowly, all corners of the nasopharynx, the region on top where the adenoid rests may be found, and the openings of the Eustachian tubes, can be examined. At the same time, the nasal cavities can be viewed from the rear, thus getting a view of the posterior structures which are difficult to see through the nostrils. For this reason, this examination is called *posterior rhinoscopy.*

Now, the moment has come for that part of the examination which, to the professional speaker or singer, culminates the checkup: the *laryngoscopy* or inspection of the larynx. To see the vocal cords and the interior of the larynx, the *laryngeal mirror* — Garcia's gift to medicine — is employed. Larger than the postrhinoscopy mirror, it is attached to the handle at an angle of about 45 degrees. Before introducing it, the doctor asks our patient to stick out his tongue and grasps it with a small piece of gauze. The gentle pull at the tongue has a twofold purpose: it draws the tongue forward, thereby widening the space between tongue and throat, and, at the same time, it helps to elevate the epiglottis, which normally overhangs the entrance into the larynx.

After a few examinations, the patient learns to do the tongue-pulling himself, thus freeing one hand of the doctor for any treatment he might want to give. Since this is our patient's first examination of the larynx, the doctor holds the patient's tongue with one hand. With the other hand, grasping the handle like a pen, the warmed mirror is guided slowly into the mouth until it leans against the soft palate. Our patient cooperates well. To his pleasant surprise, he does not feel anything because the doctor avoids carefully any touching of the throat which is much more sensitive than the palate.

From your corner, you cannot see much. Even looking over the doctor's shoulder would not help you. You would be able to see the laryngeal mirror in place, but you would look at the mirror at an oblique angle and would miss the straight view the doctor has through the hole of the head mirror. In laryngeal examination, only one person can see the vocal cords, which makes the demonstration of laryngeal patients to a group of students difficult. Since you cannot see for yourself, we had better come to your assistance with an illustration (Figure VIII-1). The light, thrown into the mouth by the head mirror hits the laryngeal mirror. From there it is reflected downward and illuminates the interior of the larynx. At the same time, the image of the larynx is caught in the circular mirror and reflected back into the eyes of

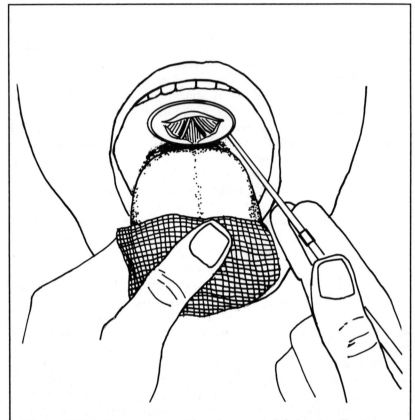

Figure VIII–1. *Laryngoscopy. The physician's left hand pulls the patient's tongue out, while the right hand introduces the laryngeal mirror, in which the image of the larnyx appears.*

the doctor behind the opening in the head mirror. The doctor *sees* the larynx.

Figure VIII–2 shows you laryngeal images as seen in the mirror. It is a kind of bird's-eye view from above. The epiglottis appears as a sickle-shaped roll (the upper rim), the arytenoid cartilages stick out as small buttons, and the vocal folds are visible as white (or pinkish white) bands in marked contrast to the red of the mucous membranes, which cover the false cords and the rest of the interior of the larynx.

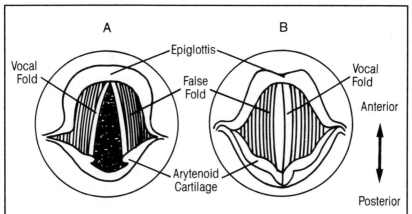

Figure VIII-2. *The larynx as seen in the laryngeal mirror.* (**A**). *The position of breathing with spread vocal folds.* (**B**). *The position of phonation with approximated vocal folds. Structures at the top of the figure are anterior in the larynx; those at the bottom are posterior.*

While the patient breathes quietly, the glottis remains open with the triangular spread of the vocal folds. Through the glottis, the upper part of the trachea with a few cartilaginous rings can be seen clearly.

To study motility and closure of the folds, the doctor asks our patient to say "ee" with a high voice. This elevates the epiglottis even more and brings the cords into the position of closure. As ingenious as this simple examination is, it has a number of limitations. Since it presents a view from above, the upper surfaces of all the laryngeal structures are visible, while other details are difficult to see or remain entirely hidden. For instance, only the upper rim of the vertical epiglottis is visible while the body of the cartilage can be observed only in glimpses. Only the flat upper surfaces with the inner edges of the vocal folds are exposed while the lower surfaces remain always hidden like the other side of the moon.

This is a serious handicap because a growth that starts at the lower surface of a fold can remain invisible and inaccessible until it envelops the rest of the fold or begins to protrude into the glottis.

Another difficulty is based on the fact that one does not observe the larynx directly but looks at the mirror image. A mirror reverses sides. As you see in Figure VIII-2, the anteriorly located epiglottis appears in the mirror on top, while the posterior part of the larynx with the wide spread of the glottis is seen at the bottom. Right and left are similarly reversed. Finally, laryngoscopy — as all examination of ear, nose and throat — is done with one eye alone. We need the stereoscopic vision of both eyes to judge depth and distances. Looking at the flat mirror image with one eye, the doctor would lose all depth perception if he were not helped by an intimate knowledge of the anatomical structures. It requires great dexterity and constant practice to overcome all of these obstacles in laryngeal examination and treatment. Using the image that appears in the mirror as his sole guide, the doctor has to learn to translate automatically the mirror observation into the correct anatomical relations.

You can demonstrate to yourself the difficulties of *indirect laryngoscopy,* as the mirror examination of the larynx is called, by a simple experiment. Put your watch on the table behind a heavy book or a small box that hides the watch from your direct observation. Then take a pocket mirror in your left hand and hold it at an angle over the table until you can see the face of the watch in it. Now close one eye, grasp a pencil with your right hand and try to touch some of the numerals guided only by what you can see in the mirror. Most likely you will have a difficult time. Everything is topsy-turvy. The 12 is at the bottom of the image, the 6 is on top, and the numerals are reversed. Even telling what time it is will not be easy. And, at least at the beginning, the point of the pencil will refuse to obey your simplest directions.

If you now realize that the doctor holds the laryngeal mirror on a long handle, that he has to direct light from the head mirror to the laryngeal mirror, and that all instruments used for treatments have to be sharply curved to follow the around-the-corner way of approach, you will understand why even the simple laryngeal examination you just witnessed is quite a feat.

*R*ecently, a new instrument, the fiberscope, has become an important addition to the medical armamentarium. It is very useful for examining patients who have a marked gag reflex that makes inspection of the vocal cords difficult. The fiberscope basically consists of a flexible bundle of hair-thin strands of fiberglass, compressed into a sheet of watertight plastic, fitted with optic lenses at both ends, and a tiny source of light at the posterior end. Instruments of this type have been used to look into hollow spaces of the body like the bladder and the intestines. It is now used to inspect the vocal cords.

The long cable, the thickness of a thin pencil, is introduced through the nose and advanced until the front end hangs over the vocal folds. The maneuver is painless because a mild local anesthetic is applied inside the nose. Because light is conducted through the hundreds of fiberglass strands in the flexible bundle, the image seen at the proximal end will travel through the bending cable, thus permitting easy observation of the vocal folds. Since the mouth is not obstructed by the instrument, this observation permits inspection of the vocal folds in actual singing and speaking. The optic cable can be connected to a movie camera or the image can be projected on the screen of a television set.

For surgical procedures, *direct laryngoscopy* is being used. By overextension of the head and a strong pressure on the tongue, it is possible to bring the mouth, the tongue, and the larynx into one straight line. In *direct laryngoscopy,* a special instrument with a kind of heavy tongue depressor on a strong handle is used. Grasping this instrument firmly by the handle, the doctor slides the tongue depressor with some degree of pressure over the tongue of the patient and guides it over the epiglottis until he has a direct view of the vocal cords. Light is furnished by a tiny bulb at the tip of the tongue depressor. Local anesthesia is necessary for this procedure. Instruments for treatment or operation can be straight, and the eye of the surgeon can control their action without the help of a mirror. Direct laryngoscopy is usually done in a hospital. It is used in the examination of patients with hard-to-see vocal folds and for operation on the folds.

At this point I should like to propose that we leave the doctor's examination room. The checkup I watched together with you was a good demonstration of the methods used in examination of the vocal organs. I hope it was sufficient to convince you that such an examination should not be faced with any apprehension. It requires great practice and skill for the doctor but on your side only confident relaxation. That should not be too difficult for you now.

I propose to devote the remainder of this chapter to the methods of *investigation of vocal function* that are used in research. Our knowledge of the human voice is a result of such studies, most of them done in the last fifty years. Their findings fill a whole library. I shall mention just a few of the more important methods.

One of the earliest and most fruitful approaches is the *study of breathing movements* in singing and speaking. While x-rays are very helpful in clarifying the movements of the chest and the diaphragm, they do not reveal much detail about air consumption. To study this, the *spirometer* has been used. The singer or speaker breathes into a mask, the air is conducted from there into a bag which is equipped with a gadget that measures the volume of collected air, while certain notes or phrases are sung or spoken. Instruments of this type are available that register the flow of outgoing air as a curve on ruled paper.

Another method, called *pneumography,* employs an indirect approach (Figure VIII–3). Inflated rubber belts are placed around the chest and the abdomen of the person to be examined. Any movement in breathing changes the air pressure in the belts, which are connected by rubber hoses to pressure-sensitive capsules. These, in turn, move pointers which write curves on the surface of a slowly revolving drum. You might have seen a similar set-up in the instruments writing curves of barometric changes. Pneumography can be used to study chest and abdominal breathing in speaking or singing of whole phrases. In a famous book publishing in 1923 Dr. M. Nadoleczny offered the results of many years of exhaustive research of all phases of artistic singing. He chose characteristic parts of arias for his investigations and produced curves which show the breathing movements of good and bad singers and lyric and dramatic voices with great clarity. The method is also valuable in the study of all kinds of abnormalities of breathing in singing and speaking and in disturbances of function of the vocal folds.

When you read the description of the vibrations of the vocal folds in Chapter II, you might have asked yourself how any knowledge of these fast movements has been obtained. In speaking or singing, the folds vibrate, depending on the pitch, at the rate of sixty to two thousand times per second. No human eye can follow individual movements that are faster than six times per second. This fact is used in cinematography where the showing of sixteen separate pictures per second are, for our eyes, blended into one continuous motion.

If we look at the vocal folds in singing with the laryngeal mirror, we do not see any motion. The folds seem to stand still in the closed position. Their vibrations are too fast for our eyes. To make them visible, an optic trick, called *stroboscopy,* can be employed. Between a strong light used for laryngoscopy and the head mirror that reflects the rays, a fast rotating disk is placed with a number of slits which permit the quick passage of stabs of light. The disk rotates on the axis of a variable-speed motor. If the slits in the disk rotate at a speed that equals the number of vibrations of the folds, the folds seem to stand still; but if we vary the speed slightly, we suddenly have the impression that the folds open and close in slow motion.

What actually happens is that each slit picks out a different phase of the fast motion of the folds. The eye of the examiner combines these single phases into one apparently slow motion. Examination with these mechanical stroboscopes was very difficult. The patient

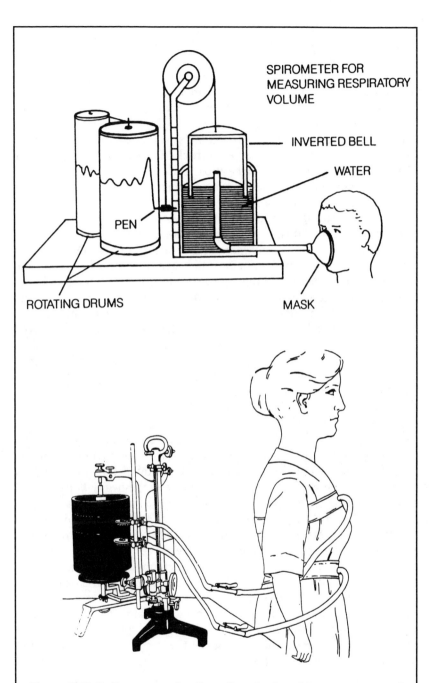

Figure VIII–3. Pneumography. Recording the breathing movements of the chest and abdomen.

had to hold one note at a very exact pitch, and the examiner had to adjust the slightly delayed or accelerated speed of the motor with the revolving disk very carefully. Modern electronic technique has made possible the construction of stroboscopes where the voice controls directly the flashes of light. The voice is picked up by a microphone circuit which automatically steers a flickering source of light at any desired accelerated or delayed ratio.

In stroboscopy, the examiner has to keep in mind that he does not see the actual movement but the results of an optical trick which might be misleading in many details. Still, stroboscopy has taught us a great deal about a hitherto invisible motion.

With the advent of *cinematography,* the goal of making vocal fold vibrations visible seemed to be within reach. But for a long time the technical difficulties could not be overcome. Aside from the handicaps that beset any cinematography of hidden regions of the body, no camera could be built which permitted the taking of pictures at the required rate. Finally, in 1940, the Bell Telephone Laboratories solved the problem by constructing a camera, which takes pictures at the fantastic rate of four thousand exposures per second. For the first time, the vibrations of the folds could be actually seen, not in the trick-slowing of stroboscopy but as actual movement.

X-rays have been used extensively in studying the breathing movements of jaw, larynx, chest, and diaphragm. To photograph the vocal folds by x-rays is very difficult because x-rays, during their passage through the body, register any resistance by heavier tissue they meet anywhere on that route. In the frontal position — which alone shows the profile of the folds clearly — the heavy bones of the spine blot out the weaker shadows produced by the folds.

Lately, a new technique of taking x-rays has been introduced. By this very ingenious method, called *tomography,* it is possible to bring a plane at any desired depth into sharp focus while omitting all structures in front or behind that plane. Tomographs are used extensively in x-rays of the lungs, where they help in determining the exact place of an infection or a growth.

The same method has been employed to obtain sharply defined x-rays of the vocal folds without the disturbing bone shadows of the spine. Excellent tomographic studies of the vocal cords in singing and speaking have been made, but the machinery is still too complicated for general use.

One of the best and most versatile tools in vocal research is the *analysis of sound.* In Chapter II we discussed the fact that pure sounds hardly exist in nature. All of the sounds we hear are a mixture of a basic frequency, the fundamental, with a number of partials, the overtones. The German physicist H. von Helmholtz was the first one to study these sound mixtures systematically. With his resonators sharply tuned to single frequencies, he could pick out all of the components of a given sound. Examinations with this methods were time-consuming and incomplete, but Helmholtz's book *Sensations of Tone,* which he wrote in 1863, remained for a long time the bible of musical acoustics.

A tool in analysis of sounds is the recording of the *sound spectrum.* This is done by so-called *wave analyzers,* which register automatically the number and the intensities of the overtones together with the fundamental. The readings produce spectrograms that provide a spectral picture of a short sample of speech or song. To the experienced eye, these sound spectra or *sound profiles* show the characteristic sound qualities of each voice or instrument at a glance. The study of such graphic recordings has supplied the answer to many acoustical questions.

Voices of different types, open or covered singing, and use of the registers can be studied and identified from their typical sound spectra. Dr. C. Culver, who has pioneered in this field, believes that the knowledge derived from these rapidly advancing investigations will deeply influence the methods of voice training. In the phoniatric laboratories that now do scientific studies of vocal function, an array of new, highly sophisticated research tools have been developed. To describe them in detail would be beyond the scope of this book.

We are still far away from a complete understanding of all the factors that go into the makings of a sound, instrumental or vocal. The teacher, the doctor, and the voice therapist have still to rely on the sensitivity of the trained ear as their finest tool. But there can be no doubt that modern acoustical research has provided us with a wealth of new information that can no longer be overlooked by anybody who is interested in the mechanics of the human voice.

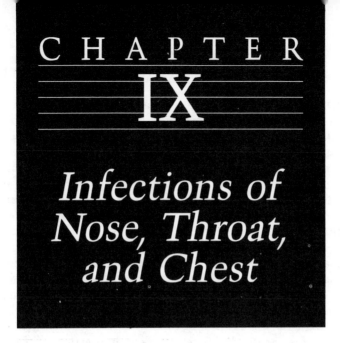

CHAPTER IX

Infections of Nose, Throat, and Chest

*A*ll vocal organs are part of the respiratory tract. The mouth and throat do additional duty as intakes for food, and the nose and mouth are the only unprotected openings in the armor that shields our body against infection. The skin, as long as it is unbroken, covers all surfaces. The few openings are carefully sealed, the ear canals by the drum, the points of elimination by muscular closure. But through nose and mouth bacteria and viruses pass easily with the inhaled air. Infections of the respiratory organs rank high in statistics of diseases.

The virus of the common cold acts as the door-opener for germs of all kinds by weakening the resistance of the mucous membranes. The primary infection by the cold virus prepares the way for secondary infections by bacterial invasion. Infections of the sinuses, the ears, the larynx, and the bronchi are, in the majority of all cases, the second stage of the war of infection against the respiratory tract. The shock troops of the invading virus are followed by the regiments of bacteria, which hold and extend the conquered positions. But it sometimes happens, too, that a host of particularly virulent germs takes over directly without previous help of the cold virus. Streptococci, for instance, may overwhelm the defenses of the throat and produce a painful tonsillitis.

Infection of any part of the respiratory tract impairs, to varying degrees, vocal function. As a matter of fact, disturbances of voice production are frequently out of proportion to the actual tissue alterations in respiratory infection. So complex and finely adjusted is the mechanism of the voice that any change in body sensations throws it out of gear. For this reason a discussion of respiratory infections is in order in a book on vocal health. Of course, I shall not attempt textbook completeness but will limit my description to conditions of special interest for the voice professional.

In discussing these infections, I will follow the same route as in our study of anatomy, beginning with the nose and sinuses, considering mouth and throat and then — skipping the larynx — descending to the trachea and bronchi. The diseases of the larynx, the most important of the vocal organs, will require a chapter — the next one — of their own.

Since this chapter deals exclusively with *infections*, a few general considerations will be useful. In medical language any infection from germs that do not cause a specific disease — such as diphtheria or whooping cough — is named by adding the ending "itis" to the affected organ. Thus we speak of sinusitis, tonsillitis, laryngitis, and bronchitis. Most respiratory infections are caused by members of the family of cocci. Streptococci are the most frequent criminals, with staphylococci and pneumococci close seconds.

To the patient, who cannot see the germs, the symptoms of the infection — such as fever, congestion, cough, and pain — are the disease itself. Actually, these symptoms are the effects of the defense of the body against the infection. Raising the temperature — the fever — creates unfavorable conditions for the multiplication of germs in the blood. Dilation of blood vessels — causing the congestion and swelling of tissues — increases the blood volume in the infected tissues and maximizes the healing forces of the blood. Pain — started by pressure of the swollen tissue on the nerve endings — makes the patient aware of the presence of an infection and forces him to rest the sick organ.

Even pus, the dreaded symptom of more severe infections, is a product of active body defense. The white blood cells, the fighters of the blood, attack the germs in the tissues, dying in the battle by the millions. Their dead bodies, together with destroyed and still living germs and the remnants of tissue cells, form pus, the scrap of antibacterial warfare.

The doctor fights the infection itself, while the patient wants to get rid of the symptoms. The doctor should not interfere with the defense mechanism of the body. Pain can be alleviated by drugs, but fever or congestion should not be reduced to the point where the self-help of the body would be endangered. Local pain may give important clues that help the doctor to judge progress or conquest of the infection. Forceful suppression of pain by powerful drugs may mask the symptoms of an expanding infection that requires surgical action. In short, the patient should always keep in mind that both body and doctor have the primary task of fighting infection, not the discomfort it causes.

All of the infections we shall now consider follow this general pattern. Their individual characteristics are determined by the special anatomical features of the affected organs. If a plain nose cold does not end in the usual short course of a few days, secondary infection may extend into one or more of the sinuses. The symptoms of *acute sinusitis* are shaped by the unique anatomical situation. The sinuses are bony cavities lined with mucous membrane which are connected with the nose by small openings. The general swelling of all mucous membranes narrows or even closes the opening of the affected sinus and interferes with the drainage of purulent discharge. The result will be increased pain, centering around the infected sinus (but sometimes "referred" to other parts of the head).

By pressing with the finger the regions of the cheek and above the eyes, the doctor gets the first indication whether one of the maxillary or frontal sinuses is infected. In maxillary sinusitis, the close proximity of the roots of the upper teeth to the floor of the sinus may produce "toothache" in the upper jaw and send the patient mistakenly to the dentist.

Next to pain, the change of nasal discharge from the glassy mucus of the cold to thick yellow pus is indicative of sinusitis. In examining the nose of the patient, the doctor watches for the telltales of pussy drainage from the sinuses. As you remember, the maxillary and frontal sinuses as well as most of the ethmoid cells drain into the middle meatus. Only the sphenoid sinus, which is least frequently affected in acute sinusitis, has its opening in the rear, near the posterior end of the middle turbinate. Pus from the other three sinuses will become visible in the middle meatus.

Of course, this symptom will help the doctor only if visible drainage exists. This is not always the case. The maxillary sinus, for instance, has its opening near the ceiling, like the overflow of a sink. Only if the whole sinus is filled with discharge will pus be drained into the middle meatus. The frontal sinus has its opening at the floor, but it is narrow and easily closed by swelling of the membranes. The ethmoid cells are a labyrinth of small cavities, interconnected by small openings. Here, too, drainage is easily interfered with.

If neither localization of pain nor observation of sinus drainage gives conclusive proof for a diagnosis, transillumination or x-rays can unveil the place of infection. If one puts a small electric bulb under the eyebrow or into the mouth, the frontal and maxillary sinuses light up with a pink glow if they are healthy and filled with air. In infection of one of these sinuses, the swelling of the mucous membranes and the retained discharge prevents the passage of light. Instead of showing translucent glow, the infected side remains dark on *transillumination*. It is a simple procedure which can be used in the darkened examination room. Its limitation is that it does not reveal anything about the condition of the ethmoid cells and the sphenoid sinuses.

For a complete check-up of the sinuses, x-rays are necessary. Infected sinuses appear in milky cloudiness on the film. Fluid levels of discharge in a sinus may be visible. X-rays of the sinuses are helpful, too, in differentiating between actual involvement of the sinuses and neuralgia, which is the painful irritation of the sensory nerves. Neuralgia of the supraorbital nerve, which emerges from the bone at the middle of the eyebrow, can produce pain that is quite similar to that of frontal sinusitis. X-rays will decide the diagnosis.

As a rule, acute sinus infections are easily diagnosed. Infections of the maxillary sinus are leading in frequency with ethmoid and frontal sinusitis next, and sphenoid sinusitis relatively rarer. All kinds of combined infections are possible.

What does sinusitis mean to the patient? There is definitely no cause for the widespread fear that sinus troubles are permanent. The vast majority of all cases of acute sinusitis are cured with the help of modern drugs, without later recurrence. On the other hand, acute sinusitis requires two things: medical help and a few days of complete rest. The latter is particularly important for the speech and voice professional. It should always be kept in mind that the whole respiratory tract is a unit. If one part is infected, the rest of the tract is always involved, even if to a lesser degree. Infections spread easily from one area of mucous membrane to others. If we speak of sinusitis or laryngitis, we mean by that term that the respiratory infection has centered around this or that part of the tract, but some degree of irritation is usually present in the rest of the respiratory system.

Complete rest creates the best conditions for fast healing of the infection at the storm center and gives the neighboring parts a chance to mobilize their resistance to approaching trouble. In the case of sinusitis, the danger of the spreading of infection to the larynx is particularly acute because of the constant downward drip of infected discharge from the sinus.

The treatment of acute sinusitis is aimed at making the patient comfortable, establishing good drainage, fighting the infection, and restoring normal function. Anything that improves drainage and reduces tissue swelling will increase the comfort of the patient. Until that is effected, pain-killing drugs may be necessary.

To restore drainage vasoconstrictors are used as drops, sprays, or packings. Since the sinus openings are hidden in deep recesses, drops and sprays applied by the patient are not sufficient. In office treatment small pledgets of cotton, saturated with a vasoconstrictor, are placed near the sinus openings and left there for a while. Frequently, this treatment, which improves sinus drainage by shrinking the mucous membranes, is combined with external heat applied by infrared lamps or similar equipment.

But the frontal attack on sinus infection is made by drugs. Due to mass publicity and to stupendous successes, antibiotics are extremely popular with patients. They clamor for the drugs and they get them all too frequently.

Ours is a civilization of waste. We waste food as never before in history, and we get vitamin deficiencies in the midst of plenty. We waste big words on the artificial excitements of advertising, and we lose our discrimination for real greatness of speech. We waste exaggerated emotions on soap operas, cheap songs, and movies; and we lose responsiveness to the finer shadings of emotional expression. We waste antibiotics — which, in other parts of the world, still demand their weight in gold to save the dying — on minor illnesses, and we get allergies and drug-fast germs.

The frequent administration of antibiotics for every minor infection is a risky procedure. It easily sets in motion the mechanism by which an allergy is produced. Such allergies are not only extremely unpleasant, but they eliminate the drug from future use in a real emergency.

Too small and too few doses are equally unadvisable. As every soldier knows, one should leave a dangerous enemy alone or kill him. In the administration of antibiotics, the fault of underdosage often lies with the patient. After one shot of penicillin, he or she feels much better the next day and decides to avoid the expense of further treatments. The germs revive after a few days and produce a dangerous relapse. Worse yet, they have learned to live with the drug; they have become penicillin-fast. The next patient who inherits the infection with such a penicillin-fast strain of germs is in a bad spot. He will show no improvement in spite of large and continuous doses of penicillin. The same behavior of germs has, of course, been observed with all other drugs of the antibiotic group.

Antibiotics should be handled as the big guns they are. They are useless in fighting common colds because they do not influence the cold virus. They should be used only in more severe infections and then in high doses and for a number of days. They should not be discontinued before *all* symptoms of the acute infection have completely disappeared. That is not for the patient to decide but for the doctor who knows what to look for.

Before penicillin, the treatment of an acute sinus infection used to be a long-drawn and rather unpleasant affair, with irrigation of the sinus being the only active procedure and too many cases ending in chronic troubles. Today, we do not touch the acutely infected sinus. We give large doses of antibiotics, take care of the drainage by sprays or painless packings, add external heat for further speed-up of healing, and make the patient comfortable by pain-killing drugs. If the patient behaves and rests for the duration of such treatment, the vast majority of acute sinus infections are cured within a few days without leaving a trace.

Chronic sinus infections, which used to trouble the lives of so many patients, are mostly the result of incomplete cures of acute infections. With the general application of antibiotic therapy they have sharply declined in number. Chronic does *not* mean incurable. Even obstinate cases are now frequently brought under control. Where a complete cure is not feasible, at least troublesome flare-ups can be successfully handled with modern therapy. In many of these cases, allergy forms the basis of the weakened resistance of the mucous membranes. Testing for allergy and treatment by elimination, allergen shots, and antihistamines (see Chapter VI) have become valuable tools in dealing with otherwise intractable chronic sinus infections.

Surgery of the sinuses — a frequent occurrence twenty years ago — is only rarely needed these days. The only operation that is still in common use is the correction of a deviated septum. If the deviation interferes with free drainage of a sinus, the removal of the obstacle by a relatively simple operation helps greatly to clear the chronic sinus infection and restore normal function.

Polyps are glassy bodies which are outgrowths of the irritated mucous membrane of the sinus. Removing them helps to re-establish nasal ventilation and sinus drainage, and may be indicated in chronic sinus infections. Sinus irrigation (washing out of the sinus) is sometimes of value in particularly stubborn cases.

Before leaving nose and sinus troubles, I would like to say a word about that favorite symptom of so many patients, the famous postnasal drip. Of all the complaints of nose and throat patients, this is the one the doctor hears most frequently. Somehow, the public has been sold on the idea that mucus in the throat is a dangerous condition that should be fought. Actually, as we have seen in Chapter I, all mucus produced by the membranes of the nose and sinuses is transported backward by ciliary action and finally wiped from the throat by the soft palate.

The pollution of the air we breathe in the cities, the irritation caused by the nasty habit of inhaling smoke and blowing it out through the nose, and many other factors stimulate the production of mucus. The result is the "drip" of mucus into the throat. This in itself is quite harmless. So is the swallowing of mucus. The stomach does not mind mucus, it produces some by its own glands. And the acidity of the stomach kills the occasional germ caught by the mucus while it was still in the nose.

The situation is different if nose or sinuses are infected. Then the drip of purulent discharge spreads infection downward to the throat, the vocal folds, and the deeper respiratory tract. If such infectious material appears in the nasopharynx or throat, the source has to be found. With the clearing of the local infection, the postnasal drip of infected mucus will stop.

T racing the infection downward, we come now to the throat. There we have a whole group of organs which have a special affinity to infections: adenoids, tonsils, and lingual tonsil. In Chapter II described these accumulations of so-called lymphoid tissue arranged in a ring with the adenoids on top, the pharyngeal tonsils on both sides, and the lingual tonsil at the bottom (see Figure I-2).

The function of these structures is still open to argument. They belong to the anatomical class of glands, which are found in all parts of the body. Glands have the task of localizing infections and of preventing the spread of germs throughout the body. The glands of the tonsillar group seem to be more important in early childhood when they help to build up general resistance to infection. The trouble with these structures is that their own ability to kill germs breaks down rather frequently. In that case they become centers or foci of infection which endanger health instead of protecting it.

The adenoids, because of their position in the nasopharynx, can cause a lot of local trouble. If they are large enough to block the rear exit of the nose, they prevent nose breathing. In addition, the proximity of adenoids to the Eustachian tubes accounts for frequent middle ear infections. In adults, for whom this book is written, large adenoids are rarely found. But if the removal of adenoids — usually together with tonsillectomy in childhood — was done incompletely, these remnants, called adenoid rests, maintain a constant drip of infected discharge. The patients suffer from frequent attacks of laryngitis or even bronchitis. Careful inspection of the nasopharynx with the postrhinoscopy mirror will reveal the presence of adenoid rests, often embedded in scar tissue. In these cases, revision of the nasopharynx under general anesthesia will produce dramatic results. After removal of all infected adenoid rests and scar pockets, the patient will suddenly be freed of the frequent infections of the larynx and windpipe. This is, of course, a particularly pleasing result to the voice professional who has suffered, sometimes for years, from this hidden focus of infection.

Fifteen or twenty years ago the pharyngeal tonsils had, at least in adults, become almost as extinct as the dodo. Parents had been taught to ask for removal of the tonsils as soon as the poor children could stand the operation. But nature, in its stubbornness, refused to take the hint. Babies continued to be born with tonsils as standard equipment.

In the meantime, the enthusiasm for tonsillectomy has abated somewhat, both with doctors and parents. More and more children are permitted to reach adulthood with the tonsils still safely in place. Most of these lucky people will go through life without ever experiencing any tonsillar trouble. During puberty, an absorption of tonsillar tissue takes place anyhow. Healthy adult tonsils are, as a rule, small and hardly visible on both sides of the tongue between the pharyngeal pillars.

Occasionally, the tonsils are subject to repeated acute infections, lose their resistance and become chronically infected. In that case, removal is in order. If the patient is a singer or otherwise uses his or her voice professionally, the question arises whether tonsillectomy will damage the voice. Before answering this question, I want to stress the point that tonsillectomy should not be done anyhow without the strictest indication. Tonsillectomy is necessary (1) if the patient has frequent attacks of acute tonsillitis, more than one in a year or regularly year after year; (2) if the patient had one attack of peritonsillar abscess (sometimes called quinsy); or (3) if disease in other parts of the body points to the tonsils as the focus of infection. One attack of acute tonsillitis is not sufficient ground for operation. With drug treatment such an attack can usually be controlled in a few days. But frequent tonsillitis at short intervals indicates that the tonsils have lost their function as protectors of the throat. Then tonsillectomy is necessary.

Peritonsillar abcess, a common occurrence in the past, is now rarely seen. Throat infections are, as a rule, treated with antibiotics before an abcess develops. Occasionally, it still happens that pus accumulates outside of the tonsil and has to be drained by incision. In that case, tonsillectomy should be done later, six to eight weeks after the drainage.

The third indication, action of the tonsils as the focus of infection, is more difficult to ascertain. Infected tonsils may look quite harmless. Size alone is not decisive. The larger part of the tonsil is buried in the surrounding tissues, and even small tonsils can be quite vicious. The doctor has to pass sentence on circumstantial evidence, which often leaves room for honest doubt. Together with the family physician, who knows more about the patient's past history, the specialist has to weigh all the facts.

Now we can come back to the question: *Is tonsillectomy dangerous to the voice?* I believe that the answer can be given in the negative, provided that a very precise technique of operation is employed. Of course, no singer, actor, or any other high-class voice professional should undergo tonsillectomy without absolute necessity. After surgery there may be a relatively short period of readjustment to the changed sensation in the throat. The voice professional should plan accordingly and leave time for this process before he or she expects top performance.

Tonsillectomy is a relatively simple operation in the hands of the expert. It is not the easy procedure it is sometimes believed to be when done by the occasional surgeon. As Dr. Robert H. Fowler put it very precisely, the purpose of tonsillectomy is to remove "the tonsil, the whole tonsil, nothing but the tonsil." The muscles that pull the soft palate downward run in the pillars that envelop the tonsils. In the tonsillectomy of the voice professional, an extra-careful dissection of the tonsil will prevent any damage to these muscles. If done with this precaution, tonsillectomy will not harm the voice.

The last member of the tonsil family is the lingual tonsil (see Figure I-2). In contrast to the adenoids and pharyngeal tonsils, which often become infected in childhood, the lingual tonsil rarely gives trouble before adulthood. Enlargement of the lingual tonsil is probably the result of frequent small infections. It is frequently seen in patients who had tonsils and adenoids removed in childhood. The lingual tonsil grows later in life to compensate for the loss of the other tonsils, and then it becomes easily infected.

The patients complain about a foreign-body sensation deep in the throat, ranging from a "hair," a scratch, a lump, to a pinprick or pain on swallowing in acute flare-ups. Examination reveals two large lumps of tonsillar tissue, deep down at the base of the tongue, touching each other in the mid-line. Sometimes, the mass is so large that it obstructs the view into the larynx.

Aside from being a source of chronic irritation, the enlarged lingual tonsil impairs the free resonance of the voice. The cushion of heavy tissue at the base of the tongue forms an obstacle that partly blocks and effectively damps the sound that emanates from the vocal folds. Persons who speak or sing with a muffled or throaty voice should always be examined for enlargement of the lingual tonsil. It is a frequently overlooked condition.

The treatment of the enlarged lingual tonsil is surgical. The removal of the masses at the base of the tongue is a relatively simple procedure which can be done with little inconvenience for the patient. The operation not only eliminates the disturbing sensations in the throat but frequently effects a remarkable improvement in the quality of the voice.

If a respiratory tract infection descends from the throat into the lower respiratory tract, it may attack the larynx or become a tracheitis, bronchitis, or, if it reaches the lungs, a pneumonia. Leaving laryngitis for the next chapter, I can be brief about the rest. In a lower respiratory infection, medical care and bed rest are necessities.

A few general remarks might be in order. The descent of infection does not always proceed in that stage-wise manner. A day or two of a cold might hardly be felt by the patient when suddenly lower respiratory infection sets in with fever, severe cough, and other local symptoms. If a deep-sitting cough develops suddenly and temperatures go up, it is high time to quit all experiments with self-treatment. The doctor should be seen to determine the localization of the infection and to use whatever drugs might be necessary.

In a milder cough from the windpipe without fever, the patient may be tempted first to try cough medicine. Cough mixtures consist of expectorants, drugs which enjoy a certain reputation for loosening the heavy mucus accumulates in the air passages. An ingredient may be added to many of the standard mixtures to calm down the irritating tickle that causes the cough.

Most of these expectorants — many of them great favorites with doctors and patients — do not stand up to critical investigation in the laboratory. Not one of them has any curative effect on the infection. At best, they stimulate the production of mucus and help to liquefy dried discharge in the trachea and bronchi. Codeine is very effective in suppressing the cough reflex, but this is desirable only to a certain extent. As I said in the beginning of this chapter, to the patient, the symptoms are the disease. Singers and other professionals are particularly anxious to suppress coughing. They are afraid the coughing might hurt their vocal folds. This is true only of the violent, hacking cough sometimes seen at the end of an acute respiratory infection. A mild effortless cough is part of the self-cleaning mechanism of the lower airways. The cough reflex with its build-up of pressure behind the closed folds and the subsequent sudden release of air helps to eject mucus from the windpipe and bronchi. Keeping the air passages free promotes faster healing and reduces the danger of further downward spread of the infection.

Cough-stopping drugs should be taken only to the extent of reducing a painful, harsh cough to occasional and effortless action. The vocal folds can stand a lot of mild coughing without harm. Laryngitis is primarily an infection and not, as a rule, the result of nonviolent coughing.

In full-fledged deep respiratory infections, the antibiotics have their rightful place. Antibiotics are very useful in fighting infections with most of the types of bacteria, but if the infection is caused by a virus, such as in the ordinary cold or in influenza, antibiotics are useless. In addition, as I mentioned earlier, the indiscriminate use of antibiotics for any respiratory infection can cause the development of strains of germs that have learned to live with antibiotics. The main thing to remember is that any extension of an acute infection below the larynx should be taken seriously. No lecture, no audition, no performance, no sermon is important enough to keep the patient from the more urgent duties of complete professional silence, rest in bed, and medical care.

I n this review of respiratory infections, I have left out, as intended, the diseases of the larynx. I shall devote the entire next chapter to the troubles of the larynx, acute and chronic ones, to infections as well as to other organic disturbances.

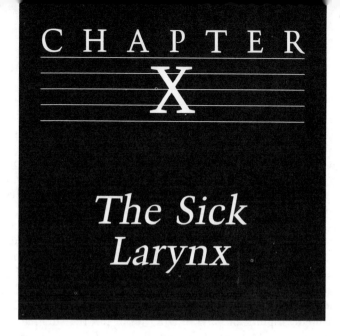

CHAPTER X

The Sick Larynx

Almost everybody knows about hoarseness from personal experience. To the average patient such an attack, if it is of short duration, is just a nuisance. But the speech or voice professional fears hoarseness as a serious handicap and a danger to the quality of his or her instrument.

Hoarseness is one of those general terms that resist concise definition. I looked up about twenty different definitions of hoarseness in textbooks and dictionaries and was shocked by the semantic carelessness and the medical incorrectness of most of them. In such a situation doctors like to hide behind a medical term. We speak of *dysphonia*, which the medical dictionaries define as any impairment of the quality of the voice.

There is a reason for this confusion. The term hoarseness covers such a multitude of different conditions that it is without value for any exact description. Besides, in the last chapter we learned to distinguish between symptom and disease. Hoarseness is an ill-defined symptom. It is the task of the doctor to find the cause of any impairment of the voice.

I will describe only those conditions that are of practical importance to the voice professional. Even with this limitation, we shall need a whole chapter for it.

*T*he most common of all dysphonias is the hoarseness in *acute laryngitis*. By now, medical terms should not impress you any more. You know that laryngitis simply means an infection of the larynx. In the vast majority of all cases, laryngitis is part of a general upper respiratory infection. Occasionally, infection attacks the vocal folds first. But, as a rule, some other parts of the respiratory tract are affected at the same time. If the nose or sinuses are involved, the drip of nasal discharge may spread infection downward to the folds; or the constant cough in an irritation of the deeper respiratory tract may weaken the resistance of the folds, which are flooded with infected mucus.

The outstanding feature of acute laryngitis is the disturbance of vocal function, which overshadows all other symptoms of the disease. If a patient has a chest cold, it does not make much difference — from a purely medical point of view — whether or not the small area of the larynx is involved. As a matter of fact, the actual degree of infection in laryngitis is, in most cases at least, relatively slight. Pain, the symptom of a more severe infection, is usually absent.

If we look at the vocal folds of a patient with acute laryngitis, we find that there are all kinds of changes, ranging from pink coloration to a deep reddening, from slight congestion to severe swelling. The latter is more important for the impairment of function than the change in color. The accumulation of body fluids in the folds, which accounts for the swelling, interferes with the free vibration of the vocal folds. Altogether, the visible changes in the vocal folds do not always correspond to the degree of hoarseness. It has been noted by many observers that very often a minor swelling and reddening of the folds produces severe disturbance of the voice.

As we have seen, the production of voice is a very complicated and finely adjusted body function that requires the teamwork of a number of organs. Any change, even a slight one, may completely upset this automatic coordination.

Dr. E. Froeschels examined the breathing of a large number of laryngitis patients with the pneumograph (see Chapter XIII). The curves he obtained revealed remarkable irregularities of breathing. Both in speaking and singing, the breathing was uneconomical and erratic during the attack of laryngitis. After healing of the infection, the breathing returned at once to the regularity of normal respiration.

These observations are interesting because they confirm the opinion, held by many authorities, that the voice disturbance in acute laryngitis often goes far beyond the immediate effect of local inflammation. Somehow, the whole apparatus of voice production is upset during an acute laryngitis. This general disturbance of vocal teamwork combines with the psychological impact of beginning hoarseness to create a situation where the voice becomes very vulnerable. As we shall see in the next chapter, many permanent voice troubles have their origins at the danger point of laryngitis.

All this is of great practical importance. It gives added significance to the first and very urgent advice given to the patient with an acute laryngitis, to keep *complete voice rest* for the duration of the infection.

Rest, as we have seen so often in these pages, is the outstanding prerequisite for fast healing of any local infection. To the professional, voice rest is essential to prevent permanent damage. The voice is not only threatened by the harm that any abuse may do to the inflamed folds. The patient must realize that he or she has temporarily lost control over the delicate teamwork of his or her vocal organs. Any attempt to overcome this lack of coordination by force may set up wrong patterns of voice production, which will persist after the acute infection is gone.

The late Richard Tauber — once of the greatest technicians of the voice in our time — once told us that, early in life, he made it a rule for himself to cancel a performance, regardless of the consequences, if he felt the slightest irritation of his vocal folds. Observing this rule in his younger years — before world-wide fame made such decisions easier — was, he believed, a major factor in preserving the brilliance and technical perfection of his voice through a long career.

The need for vocal rest is as important for the speaker as it is for the singer. As we shall see in later chapters, the damage to the speaking voice by enforced use during laryngitis may be less obvious but still lays the basis for many permanent disorders. *Complete* voice rest during laryngitis means just that. *Whispering,* as we explained in Chapter II and illustrated in Figure II-6, does *not* rest the voice. Persistent whispering of the "stage whisper" type may strain the vocal folds even more than conversational voice. Do not talk, do not whisper, and avoid alcohol and smoking (the smoke from the cigarettes of others is as bad as your own smoking). With these precautions, the laryngitis will be gone in a few days.

Since laryngitis is usually part of a general respiratory infection, the *treatment* outlined in the last chapter will take care of laryngitis too. There is little that local applications can achieve. A few drops of metholated oil, directed to the folds by a syringe or spray, give temporary relief, but frequent use of menthol irritates the larynx. External heat applied by heat lamp or short wave or direct application of inhaled hot steam is useful as in all localized infections.

Laryngitis has the nasty habit of sometimes striking suddenly and — for the professional — at most inopportune moments. What are the chances for *emergency treatment* to enable the patient to speak or sing through a few hours before retiring for the necessary rest and cure?

One hears often about somebody's "miracle treatment" that saved a performance. At the risk of debunking the glory of such achievements, I have to tell you that in our field miracles are no more performed than anywhere else in medicine. First of all, as we shall see in later chapters, not every "laryngitis" is the real thing. Stage fright, first-night jitters, audition anxieties, election nerves, and poor habits of speaking produce hoarseness that mirrors the symptoms of laryngitis. Many a sudden recovery at the appearance of a laryngologist in the dressing room goes under the heading of reassurance.

If the patient exhibits the beginning of a true laryngitis, a few things can be done. Instillation of a vasoconstrictor on the vocal folds will reduce the congestion for a short time. A few drops of a weak solution of a local anesthetic may abolish the sensation of irritation and temporarily reverse the functional upset of voice production. But no such treatment should be given without impressing very strongly on the patient that this is *not* a treatment but an emergency measure, that vocal work under such momentary help may prolong the duration of the laryngitis afterward, that all temptation to force voice should be resisted; and that complete voice rest after vocal use under such conditions is twice as necessary.

Under good care, hoarseness in laryngitis disappears in a few days. If it persists, a laryngologist should be consulted under all circumstances to determine the cause of the voice impairment. If the vocal folds do not show any growth and move freely but exhibit the symptoms of chronic irritation, we speak of *chronic laryngitis*. In this condition, the folds are congested, red, and sometimes dry with surface crusts. On phonation, they often close poorly. The voice is raucous, harsh, and frequently produced with considerable waste of air.

In chronic laryngitis, the foremost task of the doctor is to find and, if possible, remove the cause. Infections of sinuses, adenoid rests, or the bronchi may provide a constant source of irritation. Excessive smoking and drinking and prolonged exposure to dust or chemical fumes are other causes. Finally, constant abuse of the voice may lead to a condition similar to chronic laryngitis. The rock singer who shouts through every performance, the shouting auctioneer, and the bellowing top sergeant are typical examples of vocal fold damage by prolonged strain.

This occupational hoarseness furnishes an interesting example of the intimate connection between voice and personality. The professional who uses his or her voice for highly qualified and responsible tasks reacts to the slightest disorder of the vocal folds with a pronounced upset of functional and emotional balance. But the person who gets hoarse because of occupational shouting is hardly aware of it, even if his or her voice begins to sound like a calliope or a foghorn and that person would not think of seeking medical advice.

*S*o far, I have dealt only with congestion and swelling of the whole folds. If the folds are disfigured by a localized growth, we speak of a tumor. In medical parlance, any abnormal growth of tissue is called a tumor. The term covers a wide variety of growths from the harmless corn to the vicious cancer.

A benign growth is well defined in its limits, does not invade the surrounding tissues, and does not spread to other parts of the body. Such benign tumors do not endanger general health. The trouble they cause is purely local. They may cause pain as, for instance, corns do on our feet, or they may impair the function of an organ by their presence. This happens to be the case with benign tumors of the vocal folds: nodes and polyps.

Nodes of the vocal folds are still a riddle in many respects. There is not even agreement on the nature of the growths. Some doctors do not believe that the nodes are true tumors but claim they originate from obstructed mucous glands. Others have looked at them as products of chronic laryngitis. Still others have called nodes the corns of the vocal folds. To you, these arguments may not be very interesting. What *is* important to you is the fact that nodes of the vocal folds have, almost invariably, one single cause — *wrong use of the voice.* Nodes are danger signals of the first order. They indicate that something is wrong with the patient's way of speaking or singing. Nodes appear because of abuse of the voice; once they have formed, they create additional impairment of the voice by disturbing the mechanism of vocal fold closure and vibration.

The patient seeks medical advice because he or she has been experiencing voice difficulties, usually for some time. If a singer, the patient — or the teacher — may have noticed uncertainties in the attack of soft notes or sudden breaks, usually in the middle register. The actor, speaker, or teacher comes to the doctor because of hoarseness after short periods of speaking. The voice sounds breathy, uncertain in pitch, sometimes with sudden wavering.

On laryngeal examination the doctor finds — at least in most cases — little or no reddening or congestion of the folds. But on the free inner border the doctor sees the nodes — small, well-defined thickenings that jut out as pointed or rounded prominences from the otherwise straight line of the folds. Sometimes only one node has formed, but, in most cases, they sit on exactly corresponding sites of both folds so that they touch each other on phonation. They can form anywhere along the free border of the folds but, as a rule, they develop at a point where the middle and the anterior thirds of the folds meet. They vary in size from a pinhead to a split lentil.

On phonation the nodes prevent the folds from complete contact. The patient who is aware only of a difficulty in voicing is likely to use added force to overcome the obstacle. The result will be an irritation of the vocal folds quite similar to that produced by laryngitis. Such laryngitis-like changes of the folds are not the cause but the effect of the formation of nodes. And the nodes, as I said before, are the result of misuse of the voice.

Diagnosing nodes of the vocal folds creates quite a problem for the doctor. To begin with, he or she has to inform the patient of the condition of his or her folds. There are situations in medicine where a good case can be made for circumscribing a diagnosis in vague terms or even keeping the truth from the patient. Nodes definitely do not belong in this category. If the patient is a professional speaker or singer, the responsibility is too big for any softening of the truth.

Such a revelation comes to the patient as a severe shock, particularly to a singer or actor. The patient came to the doctor because of a belief that he or she was suffering from a prolonged laryngitis. Now the patient is being told that misuse of the voice is at the bottom of the trouble.

We face here a situation we shall meet many times in the next chapters. Nothing is as hard for the voice professional to accept as the fact than an impairment of his or her voice has a purely functional basis. The professional wants to hear — and may go from doctor to doctor to get the desired explanation — that he or she is the victim of an infection. Sometimes even the singing teacher resents a diagnosis of vocal abuse, which can be considered a slur upon teaching methods.

But the doctor has no choice in this matter because the only chance of undoing the damage lies with the correction of the real cause of the condition. Fortunately, the patient can be told that such a chance exists if the treatment is planned correctly. If the nodes are relatively young, they may again dissolve if the strain is taken from the vocal folds. In the beginning, the nodes are still soft, a circumscript swelling that can be reabsorbed. The older and larger they get, the more fibrous tissue is formed, making the nodes as permanent as corns.

Voice rest alone does not achieve any cure. Small nodes may disappear after a few weeks of silence, but they will reform immediately if speaking or singing is resumed with the same abusive methods that started the vicious circle. Surgery, as such, is no answer either. It may be necessary to remove large nodes by punching instruments, but new nodes will appear as soon as speaking or singing brings the old strain back to the vocal folds.

The only effective way of dealing with nodes is to group the treatment around a radical correction of all mistakes in the use of the voice. All other measures have to be subordinated to the task of removing the strain that produced the nodes. Temporary voice rest, particularly from professional voice work, may be necessary; but reconditioning the voice should be started as soon as possible.

Small nodes do not, as a rule, require surgery. There is a good chance that, with improved speaking or singing technique, the nodes will disappear. Large nodes of longer standing have to be removed. After a short period, needed for the healing of the folds, voice training has to be started.

A successful handling of the situation depends on good teamwork of:

■ The *patient* who submits to a complete overhauling of his or her speaking and singing technique;
■ The *throat specialist,* who watches the progress by periodic examinations of the vocal folds;
■ The *speech-language pathologist,* who handles the retraining of the voice with methods we shall discuss in Chapter XII. If the patient is a singer, the team will be assisted by the work of
■ The *singing teacher,* who understands the implications of the condition and plans his or her instructions in close cooperation with the doctor and therapist.

Polyps of the vocal folds are benign growths which may emerge from any part of the folds. They may sit on the fold with a broad base as reddish prominences or may be attached to the fold by a narrow "neck." They can reach the size of a cherry stone.

If a polyp originates from the underside of the fold or from the hard-to-see anterior end of the fold, it may remain undetected, even on repeated examination. It may move up and down with the breath and become visible between the folds only on forceful expiration (for instance, in coughing). In such cases the marked hoarseness which a polyp produces will alternate with clear voice, depending on the momentary position of the polyp.

There hardly exists a laryngologist who has not had the sad experience of missing the diagnosis of a laryngeal polyp which did not "show up" and of being confronted later by the finding of a colleague who was lucky enough to examine the patient at the right moment. If the doctor is philosophically inclined — any good doctor should be — he or she will not be too depressed about such a diagnostic failure.

We still do not have a completely satisfying explanation for the emergence of laryngeal polyps. But it is safe to assume that chronic irritations (such as prolonged laryngitis, excessive smoking, constant abuse of the voice) are contributing factors.

The treatment of polyps is surgical. The removal of these growths can be done by the indirect method (with laryngeal mirror and curved instruments) if the polyp is plainly visible and accessible. But most surgeons today prefer the *direct* method, performed under general anesthesia in a hospital. The patient lies flat on the operating table with the head extended so that a straight tube can be advanced over the tongue. It permits a direct inspection of the vocal folds and creates better conditions for the surgical removal of any growth.

After the operation, every effort should be made to find and eliminate all possible causes of irritation. In this connection, special attention should be paid to the voice. To illustrate my point, the owner of a very noisy factory and a mediocre actress who both habitually strained their voices (the one by shouting in the workrooms, the other by speaking on and off stage with untrained force) had polyps removed. Within a year new polyps were formed on the vocal folds of both patients. Finally persuaded of the connection between vocal abuse and polyp formation, they both underwent systematic training of the speaking voice. No troubles have been experienced since, for six years in one case and eight years in the other.

At this point, I have to say a word about malignant tumors of the larynx, of which cancer is the most important one. I do not want to scare anybody nor to create hypochondriacs. But as long as we have no drug that cures cancer, everything depends on early detection. There is no excuse for the many cases of laryngeal cancer that still come to the doctor in a late stage. *Nobody should be hoarse for more than two weeks* without having his or her vocal folds examined by a competent specialist.

We doctors witness so much human tragedy which cannot be prevented or influenced that we hate to see lives being gambled away because of negligence or indifference. Laryngeal cancer grows slowly and remains localized for some time. If the growth is still limited to a small area of a fold, the chances for cure by an operation or radiation are good. As long as it is possible to preserve the basic structure of the larynx and remove only the affected part of the vocal fold with a good margin of safety, one can save enough for vocal function. The remaining voice may be rough but is usable.

The trouble is that too many patients treat prolonged hoarseness with an amazing indifference. They would rush to the doctor if pain anywhere in the body lasted more than a day, but they take injury to their voices very casually. They seek medical attention so late that nothing short of a complete removal of the larynx has any chance of saving the life of the patient.

In that case, the patient can, at least, take some consolation from the fact that the loss of speech, entailed by the operation, is not permanent. A new voice which uses air from the esophagus can be developed by specialized training. Many of these patients learn to speak again with this voice, which is amazingly clear and audible. Lately a number of new surgical techniques have been developed that still preserve the natural structure of the larynx while removing the tumor with a safe margin.

But let me say once more: cancer of the vocal folds can and should be detected early, at a stage where chances for cure are still good and natural voice can be preserved. There is no reason to fear cancer in every simple laryngitis, but a patient with prolonged hoarseness should be seen by a laryngologist at once.

I would like to mention in passing two more possible causes of hoarseness: allergies and glandular imbalances. I discussed *allergy* in Chapter VI and have mentioned it a few times since. I can be brief and say that any general allergy of the respiratory tract may produce laryngeal symptoms too. In addition, isolated allergic hoarseness occurs more frequently than is generally assumed. If the examination of a patient with frequent spells of hoarseness exhibits a pale congestion of the vocal folds, one has to keep the possibility of an allergy in mind.

The same symptoms may be produced by a *disturbance of glandular balance.* Underfunction of the thyroid gland is an example of such a condition. Determination of the basal metabolic rate establishes the diagnosis, and the administration of the deficient hormones will correct the imbalance.

So far, we have dealt exclusively with the possible causes of hoarseness. In conclusion of this chapter I have to add a word about *aphonia,* the complete loss of voice, by paralysis of one or two of the vocal folds. The nerves which supply the folds with motion take a very unusual course. They are branches of the vagus nerve, a large nerve trunk which passes through the neck and into the chest. Instead of going directly from the vagus to the larynx, they dip first from their origin in the neck deep downward into the chest, then turn around and return all the way up to the larynx. Because of this unique pathway, they are called *recurrent nerves.* This long course makes the recurrent nerves rather vulnerable. Any pressure they might encounter, caused by swollen glands in the chest, enlarged blood vessels, or new growths, will damage the nerve and deprive the corresponding vocal fold of its motility. If a patient loses his or her voice and the examination reveals loss of movement in a fold, the search is on for localization of the damage to the recurrent nerve.

*B*eginning with the next chapter, we shall embark on the discussion of the functional disturbances of voice and speech. It is the least known, the most misunderstood, and perhaps the most important subject for anybody who uses voice and speech in his or her work.

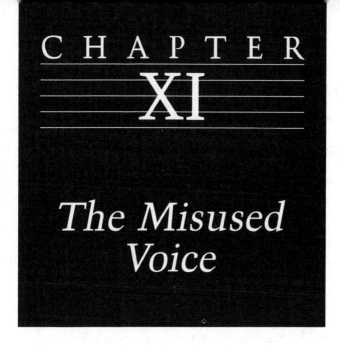

CHAPTER XI

The Misused Voice

*M*r. Smith, a high school teacher, is a worried man. For some time, he has experienced increasing difficulties with his voice.

We could call him by any other name because there are thousands like him — teachers, ministers, lawyers, politicians, salespeople, actors and actresses, and singers. They all use their voices extensively in their chosen professions. Their work is specialized, responsible, and requires a high degree of natural talent, professional training, intelligence, and authority. Voice is their great asset and, at the same time, their vulnerable spot.

Mr. Smith, whom I present as a typical example, is a good teacher who loves his work. He has an easy way with young people, his professional background is solid, his methods are modern. He is well liked by his colleagues and superiors. He is full of ambition and has good reason to assume that he is in line for the next free principalship. He knows that his superiors watch him for qualities of leadership and professional excellence. He tries hard to become a success.

But lately, he has begun to worry about the future. Slowly but irresistibly, a threat has developed to his career. It all started rather innocently. After three or four hours of teaching, his throat felt irritated, raw, and scratchy. He had to clear his throat at frequent intervals. His voice became veiled, slightly hoarse.

He attributed his difficulties to a cold and stayed at home for a day or two, treating himself with the usual home remedies. He felt fine and in good voice when he returned to his class. But a few days later, his troubles started again.

During the next few weeks, a nasty daily pattern developed. Mr. Smith woke up with a clear voice, confident that, at last, he had licked his "cold." Standing under the shower he even broke out into song. He went to school and, for an hour or two, his voice behaved well. But during the next classes, all of his difficulties returned. His throat began to burn like fire, and his voice became weak. The more he tried to overcome his vocal troubles by force, the worse he got. By the time he had reached the end of the day's schedule, he was completely exhausted, hardly able to speak above a hoarse whisper.

It never entered his mind that something could be wrong with the way he was using his voice. He had always taken his voice for granted. At college, he had learned to watch his speech. He had been told to sharpen his s, but nobody paid much attention to his voice.

When he stood in front of his first class, eager to prove himself a good teacher, he tried his best to speak with a clear and loud voice, full of energy and authority. To go through a full day of teaching was harder work than he expected. Near the end of the day one became quite tired, but that could be overcome by putting more force behind one's voice. For eight years nothing had troubled him. And now, this prolonged cold had hit him.

As a good teacher, Mr. Smith likes to rationalize the events of his life. In addition, he is a victim of the amiable weakness of his profession to fancy himself an amateur diagnostician. He has it all figured out, it is a cold and a laryngitis. What he needs is some good local treatment by a throat specialist. He goes to the doctor, tells her the story of an unusually obstinate cold, and asks for help.

The doctor, who gives him a conventional examination, has no reason to quarrel with this diagnosis. She finds the throat reddened and dry, she looks at the patient's vocal folds and discovers the congestion and reddening of a mild laryngitis. The doctor sprays Mr. Smith's vocal folds with mentholated oil, prescribes an expectorant, and recommends voice rest.

Mr. Smith feels better, goes home for a few days of rest, begins to teach again, and — is back where he started. Nothing has changed except that he has a new worry: How to pay the doctor bills for the prolonged treatment that seems to be in store for him.

If his doctor knows something about voice troubles, she will change her diagnosis at the second or third visit. She will tell Mr. Smith that nothing is wrong with his vocal organs. She will explain that the real cause of all of his troubles is a disturbance of the function of his voice and that only one treatment can help, training the voice.

If Mr. Smith is lucky, he will believe his doctor and put himself into the hands of an experienced voice therapist. Chances are that he will fight this diagnosis. He will lose valuable weeks and months, going from doctor to doctor for heat treatments, short-wave applications, inhalations, penicillin shots, and vitamin injections, getting worse all the time and slowly missing his chances of preventing the complete disintegration of his voice.

Mr. Smith might be an extreme case — although by no means a rare one — but functional voice troubles of all degrees are extremely common. To understand them I must now introduce the very important distinction between organic and functional diseases. In the second part of this book (Chapters 6-10), we dealt mostly with organic disturbances, the changes of voice caused by infections, tissue changes in the vocal organs, and new growths.

In *functional voice troubles* the primary cause of the disturbance is not a germ, a virus, or a growth, but the *incorrect use* of the otherwise healthy vocal organs.

In practice, this distinction between organic and functional disturbances is not always easy. Prolonged misuse of the voice may produce quite visible organic changes, such as the nodes of the vocal folds; or organic disease, such as laryngitis, may start the upset of function with effects that will become noticeable long after the initial infection has passed. But the term *functional disturbance* is clear enough to describe a well-defined group of voice troubles and important enough to warrant a separate discussion.

Outside of the small group of voice experts, very little is known about these disturbances. And almost nothing is done in the training of professionals to prevent slow damage to the voice by faulty use. The result is that few adults completely escape the ruinous changes from the clear voice of the average child of two or three years to the rough, shrill, throaty or breathy voice of so many adults.

If I now try to discuss with you these functional voice disturbances, I have to begin with the statement of two unfortunate limitations. Describing auditory phenomena in printed words is extremely difficult. The most important instrument of the speech-language pathologist is the ear. It takes years of training to perceive the often imperceptible changes that betray improper function of the voice. In scientific writing one can use accepted terms in the confidence that they are backed by the acoustic experience of the reader, gained through the observation of hundreds of cases. You will have to accept some of my descriptions at face value. You may be tempted — and I hope you will be — to listen to the voices around you with an improving ear for the voice irregularities you will find in abundance. With greater experience, you might even develop into quite a good judge of voices.

But you must be aware of another most undesirable limitation. If you try to judge the qualities of your own voice, you are bound to fail. Even experts are often quite unaware of the shortcomings of their own voices. We do not hear ourselves as others do. If you have ever heard a recording of your own voice, you will not forget the shock of this experience. "Is that really my voice?" asks everybody who listens for the first time to the "stranger" whom he or she hears.

The reasons for this phenomenon are both acoustical and psychological. Our ears receive our own voices and speech sounds by different channels than sounds of outside origin, and the conceptions and intentions of our brains are so strong that we may "hear" the sounds we want to produce instead of those which our vocal organs actually perform.

Having made these reservations, I can now proceed with the discussion of the types of functional voice disturbances. The voice can be damaged by using the *wrong force,* the *wrong pitch,* or the *wrong breathing.* Considering these mechanisms separately simplifies matters somewhat. As we have seen, voice is a complex process in which a number of different functions act as a unit. Disturbances of one part, at least in the majority of cases, affect the voice as a whole.

On the other hand, only the separate consideration of the single parts of the voice mechanism makes it possible to bring some order into the great variety of voice disturbances. All progress in medicine depends on the exact observation and classification of symptoms and signs of a disease. To leave this firm basis of scientific approach is to court the danger of getting lost in speculation and vague generalization.

The *wrong use of force* is the basis of most voice disturbances. In 1906, Dr. Theodor Flatau, one of the pioneers of the science of the voice, wrote a book entitled *The Functional Weakness of the Voice.* With a great wealth of observations and diagnostic detail, he described the functional voice troubles of professional speakers and singers, as a well-defined vocal disease he called *phonasthenia* (Greek for weakness of the voice). Appearing at a time when throat doctors still thought only in terms of infections and organic changes, this book marked the beginning of a new approach to vocal problems. Since then, a whole library of papers and books has been written on the mechanics and treatment of voice disturbances.

The term phonasthenia is still widely used. It is not a very good one because it describes only the last stage of functional disturbances that begin with wrong use of force and only end in weakness of the voice.

Dr. Emil Froeschels introduced a semantically more correct terminology by using the terms *hyperfunction* and *hypofunction*. *Hyper* and *hypo* are the Greek prefixes for "too much" and "too little." Hyperfunction of the voice means the use of too much muscular force — or of force at the wrong places — in the production of the voice. Hypofunction describes the weakness of the voice that occurs as the result of diminished power of the muscles of the vocal organs. The value of this terminology lies in the fact that it explains the mechanism of most vocal disturbances in a simple way. Hyper- and hypofunction are — in a vast majority of these cases — different stages of the same disorder. It begins with hyperfunction, the use of too much force. If this hyperfunction continues for some length of time, the involved muscles cannot stand the constant strain any longer, and hypofunction sets in with progressive weakness of the voice.

All of the symptoms we described in the case of Mr. Smith are only incidental to this basic mechanism. The dryness and irritation of the throat, the queer sensations in the throat and larynx which finally developed to the point of real pain, radiating even to the breastbone, and the roughness and hoarseness of the voice are but the consequences of constant speaking with hyperfunction. No wonder that all the local treatments did not help. They tried to relieve symptoms instead of attacking the disorder itself. If unchecked by vocal retraining, Mr. Smith's voice — like the voices of thousands of similar cases — will slowly go from hyperfunction to hypofunction, ending in so-called *paretic hoarseness*, the loss of all muscular power. A weak voice, breathy because of incomplete closure of the vocal folds, will be the final result.

A small group of voice disorders begins with hypofunction. This is invariably a symptom of purely psychological origin. We shall come back to this type of voice impairment when we discuss the causes of vocal disturbances.

Wrong force can be used at any part of the vocal tract. There are six locations of such hyperfunction as taught by Dr. Froeschels. The first is hyperfunction of the muscles that close the glottis. It is the *glottal stroke (coup de glotte)* which was mentioned in Chapters IV and V. The effect of the glottal stroke is the hard attack of a note in singing or of a vowel at the beginning of a word in speaking.

The second region of hyperfunction lies immediately above the vocal folds. The use of too much force there leads to *self-strangulation* of the voice. The strong contraction of the pharyngeal muscles in the lower throat creates a bottleneck, which gives the voice — both of the singer and the speaker — a characteristic constricted quality.

The third zone of disturbance lies a little higher, involving the muscles of the base of the tongue and the opposite part of the throat.

Hyperfunction there is the cause of singing or speaking that sounds as if a hot potato had gotten stuck in the throat. It gives the singing voice a rather unpleasant muffled quality, which can be heard very often in singers with a poor technique. If you listen to the voices of your friends and acquaintances for these hyperfunctions, you will be amazed at how many of them speak with glottal stroke, self-strangulation, or with the "hot potato."

The fourth location involves excessive tension of the soft palate, resulting in a flat voice without proper nasal resonance. The fifth and sixth hyperfunctions are characterized by stiffness at the tip of the tongue and of the lips. They are the result of overarticulation. Actors and singers who employ an affected manner of pronunciation are examples of this type of tenseness.

To the professional user of the speaking and singing voice, any appreciable degree of hyperfunction is a potential threat because of its tendency to accumulate and spread. Hyperfunction rarely remains localized. Sooner or later, it spreads from the point of origin until all the muscle groups of the different zones are involved. Almost all of us speak with some degree of hyperfunction; but, as a rule, this deviation from the normal, although esthetically unpleasant, constitutes no major threat to ordinary function. The fascination that the voice of a great actor or actress holds for us is, not in the least, due to the fact that — without realizing it — we are listening to one of the rare "normal" voices.

A voice specialist often can make a diagnosis by ear alone. Hyperfunction, the transitory stage of mixed function, and finally hypofunction in the various regions of the vocal tract produce quite characteristic voice qualities. The doctor who tries to examine such a patient with a tongue depressor and laryngeal mirror frequently gets his or her first inkling of the functional character of the voice disorder by the patient's behavior during the examination. Well-trained singers and speakers are, as a rule, easy to examine. Their tongues and throats are relaxed, and the folds are visualized without difficulty. Patients with hyperfunction frequently carry their habits of muscular constriction into the examination. Without intending or knowing it, they fight the examination. The tongue bulges and the throat contracts, making the observation of the vocal folds possible only in glimpses.

The folds show — at least in the first stage — very little change. As a matter of fact, the disproportion between the extent of voice impairment and the absence of any marked irritation of the folds is characteristic of most functional voice disorders. Occasionally, a red stippling of the palate and sometimes the folds, indicating tiny hemorrhages, might betray the effects of frequent use of too much force in speaking and singing. Excessive hyperfunction may lead to more extensive damage to the folds. For instance, an actor who plays a highly emotional part with uncontrolled shouting, may suddenly become quite hoarse. Laryngeal examination shows one fold with a deep-red surface, the sign of a *hemorrhage* from a ruptured small blood vessel.

In the last chapter, I discussed the *nodes* of the vocal folds. Their appearance is the result of prolonged strain on the vocal folds because of hyperfunction of the vocal organs.

In the late stages of hyperfunctional voice disorders when hypofunction takes over, the folds exhibit the growing weakness of the vocal muscles. On phonation, the folds close imperfectly, permitting the audible escape of unutilized air. This is the *waste of air* we discussed in Chapter V.

So far, we have discussed only the mechanism of the wrong use of force in vocal disorders and have neglected to discuss the *causes* of this condition. Functional voice disorders are still relatively unknown and have to be introduced first as an entity before one can deal with the "why." The mechanism of hyperfunction can be started in many ways. To begin with, we live in a tense time. Our civilization, which stresses the spirit of competition as a guiding force, transforms our lives into a constant battle for success. The general *tensing-up* that so many of us share can be traced in all parts of the body. It creates a kind of predisposition for tenseness and tightening of all muscle groups, including those of the vocal organs. The professional speaker or singer is an easy victim to vocal hypertension.

The almost complete absence of voice control and voice training in our schools is responsible for damage to countless voices during the formative years. This neglect by our schools and high schools is, too often, continued through the training for the professions that require extensive use of the voice. Young teachers, ministers, lawyers, actors and actresses who have finished their training periods and begin to work in their professions are suddenly burdened with a premature load of voice work that they are not equipped to handle. This *quantitative* strain on the voice leads to fatigue which the speaker tries to overcome with increased force.

Frequently, acute infections are the starting point of voice disorders. In the preceding chapter, we saw that in *acute laryngitis* the smooth cooperation of the vocal organs is upset, often out of proportion to the actual tissue changes. Trying to overcome a temporary handicap, the speaker or singer almost invariably uses force, and a new pattern of voice production is established that persists after the laryngitis is gone.

At this point, the deficiencies of poor vocal training combine with the effects of laryngitis to put the voice on the road to damage. The well-trained acting professional might be able to maneuver his or her voice around obstacles of acute impairment. But the professional without voice training is, at best, in good voice as long as no serious upset disturbs the automatic motion of his or her vocal organs. The difficulties of acute laryngitis throw the voice completely out of gear, and the pattern of hyperfunction takes over.

One of the causes of this problem is singing before the larynx has reached full maturity. The ambition of young students and the vanity of parents pushing to see their children perform in high school productions can ruin juvenile voices. Modern noisy music is hard enough for well-trained adult singers. Performed by adolescents, it can produce permanent damage.

Poor training plays, of course, a prominent part in the voice troubles *of the singer.* A good singing voice always achieves a maximum of tonal effect with a minimum of effort. Almost all of the unpleasant traits of poor singing are connected with the wrong use of force. Lack of natural talent, the ambition of a lyric singer to invade the dramatic field, the lure of the high voices, the drive to achieve fame in the fast-paced world of popular music, are but a few of the many factors that establish the pattern of singing with excessive force.

But more than any other cause, *emotional imbalances* of all types and degrees are responsible for the wrong use of force. The influence of momentary emotional upsets on the voice is a common experience. Under stress and excitement our vocal organs tense up, the voice becomes constricted, harsh and throaty; the pitch — as we shall see presently — goes up. Under the influence of prolonged nervous tensions, of neurotic conflicts, this pattern of constriction (the "shutting off" of the hostile outside world) settles on the vocal organs.

It is not necessary to repeat here what I said in Chapter IV about the connection between voice and personality. With the professional of the speaking and singing voice, the vocal organs are the logical place for the transformation of emotional tension into disturbances of body functions. There are countless situations that may cause and maintain this tight grip on the vocal organs. With Mr. Smith it was — among other factors — the ambition to climb the ladder to success and the fear of failure. The young minister who tries to represent authority in the face of inner immaturity and, maybe, struggles of the soul, the lawyer who pleads for a client of doubtful veracity, the politician whose existence depends on re-election, the actor in the rehearsals for his or her first important part, the singer who cannot adjust to mere moderate success — may all become victims of vocal tension. The emotional conflicts of private life — too numerous to discuss in detail — leave their mark on voices too.

An additional and important factor is the stress and anxiety *created* by the increasing impairment of the voice. A vicious circle forms. The original hyperfunction, whether more from mechanical or psychological causes, produces emotional stress which, in turn, leads to increased constriction and tightness. In sudden fear, our voices become weak, colorless, and low in pitch. Certain permanent anxieties lead to a *hypofunction* of the voice which, in such cases, is not the exhausted end-stage of tightness of the vocal organs but the direct effect of fear and anxiety. It is another form of the attitude of shrinking away from the dangers of the world, of the inhibition of addressing the next man in confident sonority.

*A*side from the wrong use of force, there are other factors in faulty voice production. *Wrong pitch* is one we have to consider. Changes of pitch under momentary emotional influences, the rise in excitement, anger, or hatred and the lowering in fear and despair have already been mentioned. Prolongation of such influences establishes the pattern of *wrong pitch* as effectively as the sequence of wrong force.

There is one time in life when a faulty pitch is established frequently. It is in adolescence with the change of voice or *mutation* which we discussed in Chapter V. Figure XI-1 illustrates *mutational voice disturbances.* The two heavy bars (D and F) stand for normal development, with the male voice descending a full octave and the female voice by one or two notes.

If the male voice does not descend but settles on an even higher level, we speak of a *persistent falsetto voice* (B). The reasons for this abnormality are not always clear. Disturbances of the balance of muscular coordination have been blamed, but it seems that emotional conflicts are the most important single factor. The boy who does not want to assume the responsibilities of adult life, who prefers to remain "mother's little boy," or who inclines to female identification winds up with this high-pitched voice, which may persist throughout life. In its extreme form, this is a very disturbing abnormality which makes the patient the constant butt of cheap jokes. While the psychological

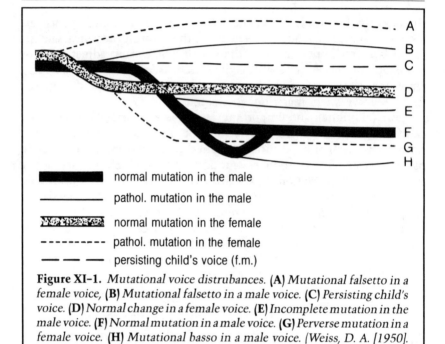

Figure XI-1. *Mutational voice distrubances. (A) Mutational falsetto in a female voice, (B) Mutational falsetto in a male voice. (C) Persisting child's voice. (D) Normal change in a female voice. (E) Incomplete mutation in the male voice. (F) Normal mutation in a male voice. (G) Perverse mutation in a female voice. (H) Mutational basso in a male voice. [Weiss, D. A. [1950]. The pubertal change of the human voice.* Journal of Phoniatics, 2, 126.]

situation that caused the disorder might be long forgotten and no longer valid, the voice disorder itself may create severe emotional tensions.

The most frequent of all mutational disturbances is *incomplete mutation* (E). The voice descends at the beginning of mutation but settles at too high a level. The result in the male voice is the pseudo-tenor, which somehow lacks firmness and masculinity. The soft Irish tenor is a good example of it. Many people speak with this voice of incomplete mutation. If they use this voice for professional purposes, they experience frequently all the symptoms of functional disturbance that we discussed at the beginning of this chapter.

More rarely, the voice descends below the level that would be normal. This is the *mutational basso* (H), the artificially deep voice, assumed, for instance, by the future preacher who wants to impress on the listener a not yet existing authority.

The mutational disturbances of women are little known, because they are less conspicuous. But they exist just the same. Perverse mutation (G), or an abnormally low female voice, may often be caused by emotional factors, such as identification with someone who has a low voice or the desire to be viewed with more authority. Voices are subject to fashions too. Imitation of the deep huskiness of famous film stars and singers has played havoc with the voices of whole classes of high-school and college girls. Lately, *mutational falsetto* with abnormally high pitch has been described in women too (Figure XI-1A).

Aside from these mutational changes, other reasons exist for assuming a wrong pitch in speaking and singing. In the singing voice, uncontrolled singing during mutation or the premature beginning of professional voice training may lead to the fixation of the voice at too high a level. All of the emotional upsets we mentioned in connection with the wrong use of force affect pitch too. As a rule, speaking at too high a level is much more frequent than the use of an artificially deep voice, for the simple reason that more situations lead to increased tension and force with the resulting rise of pitch. Imitation of and identification with individuals and groups are important factors that influence the pitch of the speaking voice.

Finally, I should mention briefly the purely organic causes of glandular disturbances (Figure XI-1C). Dysfunction or arrested development of the sex glands prevents the appearance of secondary sex characteristics and keeps the voice at the child's level (just as removal of the sex glands produced the voice of the castrate, as described in Chapter V).

The third element of voice disorders is the use of *wrong* forms of *breathing*. The functional upset of respiration has been mentioned already in our discussion of the acute laryngitis. All forms of hyper- and hypofunction involve the breathing mechanism too. In hyperfunction, breathing becomes enforced while trying to overcome the tension in the muscles of the vocal folds, throat, or tongue. In hypofunction, breathing may become shallow, with the audible escape of air between the incompletely closed folds. Of course, anything I said before about the influence of emotional stresses on the voice applies to respiration too.

Breath control is a special problem for singers. Faulty breathing is very common with singers. The trouble often starts during training of the voice. No set formula for ideal breathing fits every singer. The singing teacher who tries to impose on all pupils *one* form of breathing will only risk the ruin of promising voices. The best breath control in singing is achieved by smooth coordination of chest and abdominal breathing, and by a voice production which uses a minimum of air for a maximum of vocal effect. The preponderance of one of the breathing mechanisms is always dangerous. One of the most pernicious forms is the excessive use of chest breathing with raising of the shoulders and tightening of the neck muscles in deep inspiration. It is a danger symptom of the first order.

Faulty breathing alone or in connection with vocal hyperfunction is responsible for many cases of "off-key" singing. Control of pitch depends, to a large extent, on sensations of muscular tension. Any change of these bodily sensations disturbs the ability to find and maintain pitch at desired levels. The same consideration holds true for the speaking voice. In public speaking or acting on the stage, faulty breathing with excessive pressure frequently starts the voice disorder which, sooner or later, involves the whole vocal apparatus.

Of course, organic changes may cause similar disturbances. Allergies and bronchial asthma tighten the small bronchioles, making breathing difficult and labored. Heart failure involves the lung tissues and impairs respiration.

A last word about the total loss of voice on a purely functional basis. In the last chapter we discussed *aphonia* from organic causes. In severely neurotic persons, the conversion of neurotic tensions into physical symptoms may choose the vocal folds. The folds close well in coughing but remain open if voice is attempted. Such cases have been observed in great numbers during war when soldiers developed this type of aphonia after severe shocks. It is seen frequently in very neurotic patients. In peace time it occurs mostly in women.

In contrast to voice disorders, which develop slowly on the basis of misuse of the voice, functional aphonia almost always strikes suddenly. It is a symptom of what we used to call hysteria. The treatment of most cases is simple. All the doctor has to do is to demonstrate to the patient — by various methods of sudden surprise — that he or she can speak with a normal, loud voice. That is usually possible at the first treatment.

With the other voice disorders, it is not that easy. In this chapter, we have gone a long way from the "simple laryngitis" patients like to blame for their troubles to the rather complex mechanism of functional voice disturbances. The trouble with nature is that it is almost never simple (otherwise this chapter would be shorter). The beauty and magnificence of nature lies rather in the coordination of very complicated processes, and voice is one of the most involved functions of our bodies. By the same token, it is one of the most vulnerable ones. The treatment of voice disorders has to keep this complexity in mind. This next chapter will deal with the problems the voice therapist encounters.

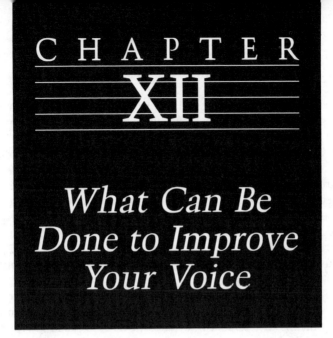

CHAPTER XII

What Can Be Done to Improve Your Voice

*I*n any medical treatment the relationship between patient and professional is a major factor, deciding, quite often, success or failure.

In organic disease the situation is relatively simple, if the diagnosis is not in doubt and the treatment promising. Patients come to the doctor with pain or other symptoms which plague them. They receive a convincing explanation of their troubles, together with a plan for a therapy that moves along conventional lines. Patients might not understand all the details but, at least, they are on familiar ground.

In functional disorders of the speaking or singing voice, no such simple pattern exists. As we have seen in the preceding chapter, the diagnosis may be perplexing to the patient. The treatment, as we shall see presently, is radically different from the drugs or surgery used in organic disease.

Even more important, in functional voice disorders, the simple patient–doctor relationship is replaced by the teamwork of a number of persons, including the patient, the doctor, the speech-language pathologist, and often the singing teacher. In some cases, a mental health professional may also be involved. In view of the importance of a clear understanding of the tasks of the members of this team, I would like to discuss their work first before taking up the methods of treatment.

First and foremost stands the *patient*. As a rule, he or she is deeply troubled by the announcement that not organic disease but rather the faulty use of the voice is responsible for the trouble. This requires a way of thinking quite different from the usual attitude of a patient with organic disease. This patient has to realize that no drug, no surgery, no local application will help, and that a complete training of the voice will be necessary.

This type of treatment requires time. Success depends, to a large extent, on the patience, persistence, and energy of the patient. Voice training means to establish new patterns of voice production. It takes weeks and often months to form and secure such new habits.

As a rule, the diagnosis of a functional voice disorder is made by the *doctor*. Deficiencies of speech are frequently spotted by parents, school teachers, and college instructors, but the troubles of the voice are usually discovered when the patient consults the throat specialist. The throat specialist should be able to differentiate the functional voice disorders from those which have an organic basis. While this is relatively easy in very characteristic or more advanced disorders, it requires a great deal of experience to diagnose functional disturbances in less obvious forms.

Since doctors like technical terms, the specialty of treating speech and voice disorders acquired a Greek name, or rather two, *phoniatry* and *logopedics*. I mention them because you might come across these terms in books and articles. If you do not memorize them, it is just as well. All of these terms look impressive on diplomas, but otherwise plain English will do quite nicely.

In the last half century, the study and treatment of voice and speech disorders became separated from the medical profession. Many colleges and universities now have communication disorders departments where a steadily growing number of professionals are trained. The great advantage of this development lies in the popularization of a new profession. Every year a considerable number of new clinicians become available in speech centers and private practices to take care of the thousands of patients in need of treatment. On the other hand, the separation of the field from medicine has deprived voice and speech therapy of easy access to some of the aspects which only a medical background can give. It has led to a certain neglect of voice problems in favor of the treatment of speech and language defects.

The blame lies mostly with the laryngologists. Too few physicians are still actively interested in voice and speech therapy while the profession of speech-language pathology has grown by leaps and bounds. By 1987 the American Speech–Language–Hearing Association, the national organization of speech-language pathologists and audiologists, had close to 50,000 members, of which only about two dozen were laryngologists. It would be most desirable for more of the younger medical specialists to join the ranks of their non-medical colleagues in the study of the problems of the human voice.

If a throat specialist makes a diagnosis of a functional voice disturbance, he has to decide whether he has enough experience to take over the treatment of the case. If not, the doctor will usually be able to recommend a good therapist to his patient. If the patient has no such guidance, he may have some difficulty in finding a therapist. The American Speech–Language–Hearing Assoication (at 10801 Rockville Pike, Rockville, MD 20852) is able to recommend individual therapists or clinics from its list of members.

While the physician and the speech-language pathologist appear on the scene only after voice troubles have begun, the *singing teacher* is already there. Choosing a good singing teacher is of utmost importance to the young singer who embarks on an artistic career. Successful growth or ruin of the voice may result from this decision. Still, it is astonishing to see how often a singing teacher is chosen in a very casual way. Judging the qualities of a singing teacher is, of course, a very difficult task. The student tends to be influenced in his or her choice by big names, either by the fame of the teacher as a singer or by the brilliant success of a student who was trained by a certain teacher.

Both recommendations are, as such, poor yardsticks of the competence of a teacher. Some famous singers have become great teachers, but not because of their artistic triumphs. Teaching an art is a task that requires abilities and experiences quite different from those needed in active performing. The great artist is often a poor teacher who forces his or her own technique on the student, which might be excellent for one singer and disastrous for another. By the same token, the choice of a teacher by relying on the big name of a famous student cannot be recommended. Some singers float from teacher to teacher. If they finally become famous, the glory of their training is in great demand. One sometimes feels reminded of the seven Greek cities which, according to tradition, fought for the claim to be the birthplace of Homer.

The good singing teacher is, first and last, someone with true abilities, which are rather rare. He or she has to have the true teacher's instinct, backed by thorough training and wide experience, of adapting methods to individual characteristics, physical and mental, of each new student. The good teacher has to be a first-class musician. And he or she has to know enough about the technique, the mechanics, the acoustics, and the psychology of singing to build his or her teaching methods on a firm basis of modern science.

The success of a teacher with a large number of different students is probably the best recommendation. The average quality of many good students with all types of voices and personalities counts more than the lucky single star pupil.

The poor qualifications of too many teachers have worried the profession for a long time. The *National Association of Teachers of Singing* has worked hard to raise the standards of teaching. Its requirements for membership are high. As of 1987, 4,600 singing teachers had been admitted. The eight districts and a large number of local branches of the Association offer to their members opportunities for study through lectures and workshops which present the advances of science and teaching practice. If local advice in the choice of a good singing teacher is unobtainable, the secretary of the Association will furnish the inquirer with a list of members in a particular area.

If a singer develops voice troubles, close cooperation between singing teacher and doctor or therapist is of utmost importance. The successful handling of functional voice disorders in singers depends on this teamwork, which is frequently missing. Doctors often know too little about the special problems of singing, and the singing teachers frequently resent any interference into what they consider their proper domain. Too often, speech-language pathologists are not much help either. As a rule, they are well trained to handle problems or defects of the speaking voice, but training in handling disorders of the singing voice is often neglected.

Very often, the doctors find themselves in a difficult spot. They may suspect that poor teaching is a major factor in the development of a voice disturbance but hesitate, for obvious reasons, to say so. Handling such situations successfully without offending the patient and antagonizing the teacher is excellent training for a diplomatic career.

The singing teacher should know that in many functional disorders special treatment is needed before regular voice training can be safely resumed. The more each member of the team knows about the field of the other, the better the chances of the patient are for complete recovery.

---

*E*motional problems and conflicts play an important part in the development of voice disorders. What help can psychotherapy give in the treatment of these conditions?

A simple answer can be given only for the relatively small group of cases where the voice disturbance is merely a symptom of a severe neurosis or a psychosis. These cases clearly belong in the hands of a mental health professional. However the vast majority of voice disorders contain both mechanical and psychological elements in varying mixtures, from preponderantly technical misuse of the voice with rather superficial emotional implications to disturbances with a decidedly neurotic or even psychotic basis. Although in many cases consultation with a psychotherapist would ideally be helpful, many psychotherapists lack the experience which is needed to judge and control disorders of voice and speech.

Finally, psychotherapy does not always provide the answer to the problems of the voice. Successful removal of the emotional conflict that started the pattern of voice disorders does not automatically correct the pattern of misuse, which has become firmly established. Personal preference and the conviction of the speech-language pathologist will decide whether the treatment of a given case should be planned around the correction of the misuse of the voice or be based on an attempt to evaluate and influence the psychological basis. The majority of cases will respond quite satisfactorily to a technical approach. As a rule, the professional singer or speaker is better off if his or her vocal function is made as independent as possible of personal emotional experience. It is preferable — and usually feasible — to break into the vicious circle of psychologically caused voice disorder from the side of the voice. In addition, voice therapy has very often a definite psychotherapeutic effect. It is fascinating to note the marked change in personality which frequently develops as a by-product of an improved use of the voice.

Of course, any good therapist will note the psychological background of a given case. Where therapists disagree is on the question of what use should be made of such insight into the emotional undertow of a voice disorder. Keeping such knowledge from the patient during a treatment does not mean to deny the importance of the emotional factor. In disturbances of a body function as personal as the voice, any kind of treatment contains a strong psychotherapeutic element. In the last resort, it is the personality of the therapist that decides the success of treatment.

---

*I*s self-treatment of voice disorders possible? Only to a very limited extent. The most important step in any voice treatment is to come to a correct diagnosis. We have seen that, because of the inability to judge their own voices objectively, patients need outside expert help in being made aware of the troubles that beset them. The same holds true of treatment.

All of the well-meaning formulas for acquiring a "pleasant" or "strong" voice that we read so often in articles and books fail to take notice of the dangers and grave risks that self-doctoring of the voice implies.

On the other hand, the goal of any sound voice treatment must be to let the patient stand on his or her own feet as soon as possible. A treatment that does not achieve this defeats its own purpose. But the reconditioning of the voice is a process that cannot be completed in a few easy lessons. The longer the misuse of the voice has been going on, the harder it will be to break the faulty patterns and to guide the voice back to normalized production.

If one believed the teachings of many of the popular books on speaking and singing, all that is needed is to learn how to "relax" or "reduce stress." Few words have lost so much of their meaning by constant and uncritical overuse. If I had my way, I would recommend to Congress the passing of a law forbidding the use of these words for a few years.

In our supercharged civilization, people try so hard to relax that they become tense all over. Using our vocal organs for the production of voice and speech is an *active* function of the body. Any action of muscles is based on varying degrees of tension (or tonus as the physiologists call it). The secret of normal function is not relaxation (which is complete only in death) but the use of the *right* muscles and the application of the *right* degree of muscle tone.

Since the majority of voice troubles results from exaggerated muscle activity, the first duty of the therapist is to see that this hyperfunction is reduced. This can be achieved by attacking the local symptoms or by dealing with vocal function as a unit. A very useful procedure to overcome stiffness of the jaw, strangulating tightness of the throat and tongue, is the so-called *shaking of the jaw*, which has become an accepted exercise with many singing teachers. While the mouth is kept slightly open and a voice sound produced, the jaw is moved loosely and rapidly from side to side. If done correctly this exercise goes a long way in breaking up the grip of tightness on the voice.

Local manipulations, as recommended by some teachers, should be avoided. They only create new hyperfunctions, which may be more dangerous than the troubles they are supposed to overcome. An exception to this rule is the application of pressure on the thyroid cartilage, which is sometimes used to suddenly lower the pitch of a high speaking voice. Pressing with the finger on the cartilage with a slight backward-downward push reduces the tension of the vocal folds and brings the voice level down. It is used only as an initial procedure to demonstrate to the patient his or her ability to speak with a lower voice. Once the purpose has been achieved, the patient is taught to speak in a normal voice without such artificial help.

Various methods have been used to strengthen muscular action in marked *hypofunction* of the voice. A weak *faradic current* passes through the neck at the height of the vocal folds raises the pitch of a given sound. Complicated machines have been constructed to combine the effect of the electric current with the tuning-up stimulation of massage. Vibration massage has been synchronized with the vibrations of the vocal folds. While helpful in some cases, it is hard to determine how much of the result achieved is due to the physical therapy and how much to the psychological impact of an impressive gadget.

In marked hypofunction or in loss of the voice (*aphonia*), due to damage to the recurrent nerve, the pushing exercises are very effective. They are based on the fact that sudden tensing of the muscles that move the arm downward stimulates the tonus of the vocal muscles too. The fists are brought down from the chest — at the height of the nipples — in a forceful manner while, at the same time, a vowel preceded by a consonant is voiced (for instance, P-Ah, P-A, P-O). Perfect synchronization between the push and the voicing is important. The method is being used in the treatment of many forms of muscular weakness: to strengthen palatal action in hypernasality, to normalize the voice in hypofunction, and to stimulate lost motion of vocal folds.

All of the commonly used methods to try to correct a faulty use of the voice by some kind of specialized exercise have a common disadvantage. They focus the attention of the patient on the part of the vocal tract around which the disturbance centers, make the patient overly conscious of the sensations and tensions in these regions. This is the common mistake of such recommendations as dropping the jaw, flattening the tongue, and directing the tone to certain parts of the vocal tract. All of these methods are based on the misconception that a "normal" pattern of positions or motions that fits every voice can be established. A treatment that would restore vocal health without paying conscious attention to single elements of voice production would be superior to all forms of such "exercise." Such an approach was introduced by Dr. Emil Froeschels, who based his treatment of voice disorders and, as we shall see, of some speech defects on the use of chewing. The function of *chewing* is a twin of speaking. We use the same muscles in chewing and speaking. Moreover — and this makes it a unique phenomenon — we can speak and chew at the same time. Froeschels believed that human speech developed out of chewing noises. Of course, no positive proof can be obtained for any explanation of a body function that emerged long before recorded history. But it seems that, thousands of years ago, the dim memory of a common origin of both functions was still alive. In the hieroglyphic script of the old Egyptians the same picture-sign was used both for speaking and eating, a kneeling person pointing at his or her mouth.

Even in pronounced disturbances of the voice the smoothness and ease of the chewing movements is preserved. In using the motion of chewing for voice production, the therapist appeals to an inborn function, which transfers the undisturbed muscular teamwork of chewing to the motions of voiced speech. Chewing consists of more than the chopping up-and-down movements of the jaw. The tongue moves continuously in a completely irregular patterns. X-ray films of chewing have demonstrated that all of the muscles, down to the larynx, are involved in an easy rhythm of flowing motion.

In a typical treatment, the patient is asked to chew the air while humming, first with the mouth closed and then open. Done correctly, a great variety of sounds can be heard. People who listen to a recording of such voiced chewing done by another person almost invariably have the impression of being confronted with a strange language. Slowly, words and whole sentences are added to this voiced chewing, and finally, the whole process is tuned down to a neutral image of chewing that can be carried over into speaking in normal situations. Since the formation of a new pattern requires constant repetition, the patient is instructed to practice chewing at least twenty times daily for a few seconds each time. The method has been used by a number of famous actors, singers, preachers and teachers with very good results.

The effect of the first correct chewing on the character of the voice is sometimes startling. The constricted voice of hyperfunction gives way to a free voice production of pleasant character. One has the impression that the normal voice has been restored by a natural process.

A similar effect can be observed on the pitch of speaking. Changing the too-high or too-low pitch of a patient is not difficult for the experienced therapist. The problem is only at what level the pitch should be considered normal. To leave this decision to the subjective preference of the therapist is a risky procedure. Chewing is a valuable aid in establishing the natural level of a speaking voice. Under the effect of correct chewing, the voice rises or descends until it has "found home."

The great advantage of the chewing method is that it activates an easily available and always undisturbed function. In using this approach, the patient bypasses the communicative character of speech and returns to vocal play, the earliest form of vocal activity. Instead of focussing on details of vocal production as all conventional exercises do, it preserves the totality of vocal function in an holistic approach.

Chewing can also be used effectively to train economy of expiration. While chewing with the voice, the client is told to "shovel" air back into the mouth with the hands. The client should have the feeling that the air flow is reversed. This is simpler than it sounds. The client who used to breathe wastefully perceives the sudden slowing down of expiration with the sensation of a standstill or even the reverse of the air stream.

An even more impressive way of achieving such an effect is to go through the pantomime of eating spaghetti. Everybody remembers that persistent single strand of spaghetti that always hangs down from the mouth and has to be sucked in by strong movements of the lips (Charlie Chaplin used it once in an unforgettable scene where he mistakes a hanging-down paper streamer for his spaghetti and goes on eating it for minutes with dreamy delight). "Eating" air like spaghetti with appropriate motions of hands and lips leads even poor breathers to perfect expiration of a slow and steady stream of air.

While such exercises, which treat the breathing act as a unit, are generally preferable, it is often necessary to strengthen neglected parts of the breathing mechanism, particularly lower chest and abdominal breathing. The main thing to remember is that lower chest and abdominal breathing should, in the end, always be a concerted function, acting as a unit. While there is a "wrong" way of breathing that should be avoided (upper chest breathing with lifting of the shoulders for instance), there is no one single "right" way to breathe. No two persons breathe completely alike, and no rigid system of breathing should be taught as a standard method. Similarly, no single method of rehabilitation of the speaking or singing voice is a panacea that helps everybody. There are many ways disturbed voices can be nursed back to vocal health, but the goal of vocal rehabilitation always remains the same. As I sometimes explain to my patients, the human voice requires the opposite philosophy of business. The less investment is made, the bigger will be the return. Most patients with voice problems suffer from "overinvestment," too much effort, too much force. In all of the details of vocal production, the minimum is always the optimum. The more economy, the better the result.

In conclusion, a word about the chances of success of voice therapy. Success depends on the degree and duration of the disorder and, to a certain extent, on the age of the patient. The earlier the misuse of the voice is diagnosed and correction is begun, the better the results. The younger the patient, the easier the transition to habits of speaking and singing. In voice disorders of patients with high-quality tasks, such as singers and actors, everything depends on early diagnosis of a developing threat to the voice. Once the voice has begun to "crack," the chances for full recovery to professional use are doubtful.

With all patients, prevention is worth more than the finest diagnosis; and early treatment is more promising than an attack on a fully developed disorder.

In a way, the work of the speech-language pathologist resembles that of the restorer of fine paintings, who cannot make a Rembrandt out of a second-rate picture, but who can very often restore some of the original beauty a painting had when it left the hands of its creator. The canvases the restorer works with show the wear and tear of time. The colors have suffered; scratches and cracks have developed; vanity has added "improvements" with new layers of paint; prudery applied a fig leaf; misguided industry contributed the false brilliance of varnish. Patiently, the restorer works, removing useless paint here, adding a stroke with the brush there. Often there is success; sometimes a beauty which was not even suspected emerges; occasionally the restorer fails altogether.

The human voice is such a work of art. The less one changes it, the more one respects and restores its original structure, the finer the result. The best therapy is one that restores as much as possible of the original beauty of a wonderful instrument.

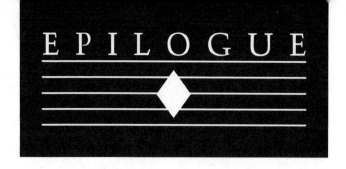

EPILOGUE

Custom has it that the author of a book on a scientific subject should speak to the reader only through the medium of the facts he or she presents. A doctor who writes for lay readers stands somewhere between the scientist and the professional writer, and may be forgiven for a personal word of parting.

I face with regret the ending of the quiet hours of writing. In our civilization, which abounds with so much loneliness in the midst of crowds, writing is one of the few pursuits where a man may be alone without being lonely. While writing this book, I was in your company. In my imagination, you became a good friend with whom I could talk things over, without hurry and hesitation, in frankness and fellowship. I hope that our conversations were profitable for you. They certainly were for me. Having gone back to many of the sources I studied through the years, I have acquired a fresh overall view of my field.

As for you, I am reasonably sure that this book will be of practical use, making it easier for you to give better care to your voice, in health as well as in disease. Beyond that, I hope that you will lay this book aside with deep admiration for the genius of creation that produced the wonderful instrument of the human voice, which is equally suited to mirror all the human emotions in song and to express the richness of the mind in speech. Essentially, both song and speech are nothing but sounding breath. The rhythm of breathing that sustains life from birth to the hour of death becomes, through song and speech, a precious achievement that lifts human beings high over all other forms of organic life.

With this instinct of a great poet, Göethe choose the tidal rhythm of breathing as a symbol of man's indebtedness to life and creator:

> Two graces are given us while we breathe:
> To take in air, to unload it with ease.
> The one oppresses, the other relieves;
> Life so wondrous a mixture achieves.
> You thank the Lord for pressure and strain,
> And thank him when he releases you again.

Subject Index